Train Your Fascia, Tone Your Body

DIVO MUELLER | KARIN HERTZER

TRAIN YOUR
FASCIA
TONE YOUR BODY

THE SUCCESSFUL METHOD TO
FORM FIRM CONNECTIVE TISSUE

- Reduce Cellulite
- Eliminate Bat Wings & a Flabby Bottom
- Get a Slender Shape

Meyer & Meyer Sport

Original title: *Training für die Faszien*

© Südwest Verlag, a Random House, Inc. company, 2015, Munich, Germany

Translated by: AAA Translation, St. Louis, Missouri

British Library Cataloguing in Publication Data

A catalogue record for this book is available from the British Library

Train Your Fascia, Tone Your Body

Maidenhead: Meyer & Meyer Sport (UK) Ltd., 2017

ISBN: 978-1-78255-117-1

© 2017 by Meyer & Meyer Sport (UK) Ltd.

Aachen, Auckland, Beirut, Cairo, Cape Town, Dubai, Hägendorf, Hong Kong, Indianapolis, Manila, New Delhi, Singapore, Sydney, Tehran, Vienna

 Member of the World Sport Publishers' Association (WSPA)

Manufacturing: Print Consult GmbH, Munich, Germany

ISBN: 978-1-78255-117-1

Email: info@m-m-sports.com

www.m-m-sports.com

Contents

Preface...8

THEORY
Let's Discover the Fascinating Fascia!... 10

CHAPTER 1
Fascia: The Forgotten Organ 12

Fascia: The Whole-Body Network 14
A Tight Skin Is More Important Than Lots of Filler 18
The 7 Most Important Fascia Chains...20

CHAPTER 2
Ingenious Tissue Architecture..24

Stress Promotes Hardening of the Fascia 28
The Two Sides of Fascial Viscoelasticity..29
Evolutionary Biology 31
Conclusion on Fascia Training 39
Test: Are You a Temple Dancer Type? 42
Test: Are You a Crossover Type? 44

CHAPTER 3
Connective Tissue, Water, and Fluid Dynamics.............................46

New Information on a Well-Known Topic: Water...............................49
Fibers, Fluid, and Cells...51
Self-Treatment: Foam Roller...54
Self-Treatment: Cupping Therapy...55

CHAPTER 4
Show Me Your Connective Tissue and I'll Tell You Your Age 58

Couch Potatoes..61
Human Species-Appropriate Movement 65
Connective Tissue Nourishment..70

PRACTICE
Fascia Training 80

CHAPTER 5
What Is the Best Way to Train the Fascia?...............................82

Tools for Fascia Training..84
Basics of Fascia Training 86
Viking and Temple Dancer Dos and Don'ts 95
The Success Formula for Healthy and Firm Connective Tissue...............95
The Basic Positions 99
Training Recommendations for Practice.......................... 102
    Shoulder-Elbow Chain..104
    Chest-Biceps Chain 112
    Abdominal Network: Straight, Oblique, and Transverse Abdominal Muscles 120
    Diagonal Lat-Glutes Muscle Chain 128
    Plantar Fascia-Heel Pad-Achilles Tendon Chain.......................134
    Foot Arch-Adductors-Pelvic Floor Chain 142
    Cellulite Special: The Fascia Lata 150
The Building-Block Principle...167

Tools and Tips..176

Acknowledgments...178

Index 179

Credits 182

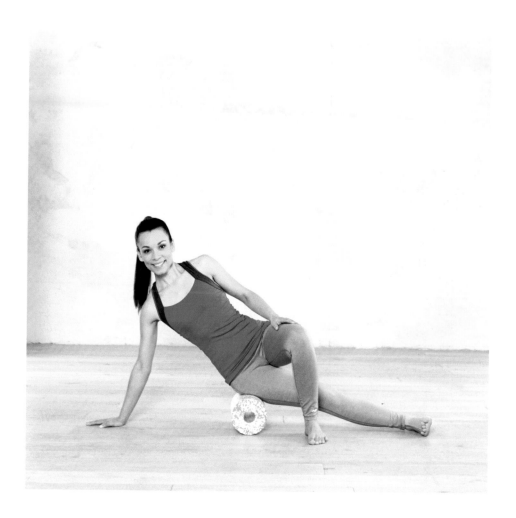

Preface

Dear Readers,

Welcome to the fascinating world of fascia, and welcome to this innovative training to create firm connective tissue. Karin Hertzer, Robert Schleip, PhD, and myself look forward to sharing our excitement for this Cinderella organ with you.

In this book we have compiled content, concepts, and new scientific findings that focus specifically on toning and strengthening the connective tissue. This book is therefore directed at people who suffer from soft, so-called weak connective tissue, hypermobility, and cellulite. There are currently several publications on the German book market featuring basic fascia training exercises that primarily focus on fostering resilience and flexibility. Most of these fascia-oriented programs were inspired by the fascial fitness training approach that we as the core team of sport scientists, fitness coaches, and physical therapists developed in close cooperation with the Fascia Research Group in Ulm, Germany under the direction of Robert Schleip, PhD.

This book has a different—and specific—goal since it focuses on strengthening the tonicity of fascial tissue and thereby improving the body's contour and definition. In the theoretical part of the book you will learn about the huge extent to which fascial tissues contribute to healthy tone. For a greater understanding we provide actual findings of fascia research in text that is easy to follow and includes lively examples.

Let us take you into the fascinating world of fascia! You will better understand your body, learn which connective tissue type you are by taking the self-test, and achieve optimal results using the training program we introduce in the second part of the book.

The subject of strengthening and toning connective tissue seems to appeal more to the female clientele. Not much of a surprise, considering nature has equipped women with rather soft and floppy tissues (without which they couldn't carry babies and give birth). Aging and the effects of gravity also take a toll, but we don't have to take that lying down. The content and exercises in this book are therefore directed specifically at women whose connective tissue is too soft and their muscles too slack. There are plenty of vicious terms for this, from flub to Jell-O to cottage cheese. Even I use one or the other in this book, but please don't take that the wrong way. Since I, as a mature women in my mid-50s, am a member of that species I dare to do so with just a pinch of humor.

The nice thing about this specific fascia training is that not only are the exercises extremely effective in sculpting the body, tightening muscles, and improving cellulite, but they are also fun. The women in my classes love the dynamic exercises, the energy of the power sounds, and the physical challenge, and not least of all, they like the all-around sense of well-being at the end of a session.

Enjoy reading the theoretical part of the book and implementing the exercises. And remember, it is not so much about dogged ambition and achieving perfection, but rather about creating a strong, elastic, and firm fascial body!

Munich, Germany, July 2015

Divo Mueller

THEORY

Let's Discover the Fascinating Fascia!

In this theoretical part of the book you can expect to find current concepts from international fascia research that has discovered and rediscovered the importance of this previously neglected tissue.

First, we will address some basic questions, and outline what exactly a fascia is and what impressive contributions this whole-body network makes to our well-being, our ability to move, and the body's contour.

Here we will primarily focus on the weak, flaccid, or too soft connective tissue types and provide background knowledge, scientific findings, and information that will help you figure out how to move through life with a toned and shapely body.

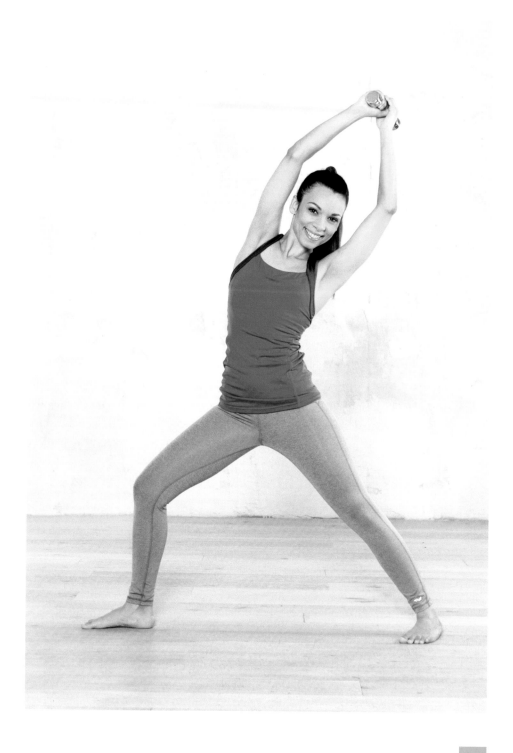

1 Fascia: The Forgotten Organ

Until just a few years ago, only insiders were familiar with the fascia. Next to a few alternative manual therapists and some proverbial die-hard scientists only the meat industry was interested in that fibrous white stuff. After all, tender meat sells better than tough.

Tender or tough, this question is essentially settled on the intramuscular connective tissue. A smaller group of chiropractors, led by the osteopaths, were already aware of muscular connective tissue in the last century. The forefather of osteopathy, Andrew Taylor Still (1828-1917), had already attributed exceptional properties and profound importance for healing to the fascia. It was, however, completely intuitive since his knowledge was not founded on a specific scientific basis. From there, Dr. Ida Rolf, an American biochemist, developed Rolfing, a deep-tissue massage, which inspired manual therapists to apply myofascial techniques with remarkable healing effects. Still, from today's point of view, the explanatory models used were outdated and not very convincing.

Meanwhile, there is a worldwide pioneering spirit. Since the first international Fascia Research Congress in 2007, held at the prestigious Harvard Medical School in Boston, the topic of fascia has become fashionable. This field is led by pioneers and mavericks, such as the young up-and-coming anatomy professor Carla Stecco (Padua University), who just recently published the first fascia anatomy atlas in medical history; the leading fascia researcher Dr. Helen Langevin (Harvard Medical School), who ascertained, among other things, that the effects of acupuncture can also be attributed to the stimulation of the collagen fibers and cells that produce collagen, the fibroblasts; and the later-in-life researcher Robert Schleip, PhD, (Fascia Research Group, Ulm University), who began his career as a psychologist and physical therapist (Rolfer and Feldenkrais instructor) and has now become an international networker for all things fascia.

Many findings from current research attest to the old intuitive knowledge, and thus the findings by Andrew Taylor Still and his colleagues that were based on dubious gut feelings. Some things must be qualified and newly evaluated from today's point of view. But beyond that the tissue that was previously neglected as relatively worthless fill-material by medical research is leading us into uncharted territory. More and more, this connective fibrous network and its liquid antagonist, the ground substance, turn out to be a jack-of-all-trades team that can be found in every nook and cranny of the body. Not only is fascia a part of the human body's every movement but it appears to also be responsible for many disorders such as chronic back pain and many other soft-tissue problems. It directly interacts with the autonomic nervous system and is sensitive to stress. In addition, it appears to be our largest sensory organ for body awareness. A current hopeful lead even suggests that the occurrence of cancer may also be linked to this matrix of life, which may result in new forms of treatments.

More diligent and sound research is needed. But one thing is already apparent: this previously denigrated-as-makeshift tissue is currently on a triumphal march with sweeping significance to exercise, health, and therapy. Modern research techniques make this possible, and the age of the connective tissue has come.

From Cinderella organ to the limelight

The whole body network is one of the most underestimated tissues in our body. Current research proves that the fascia forms an important basis for physical health and athletic performance ability. Scientific discoveries by international fascia researchers are generating groundbreaking findings, resulting in a reorientation of sports performance and medical rehab.

This also applies to all exercise programs that focus on health and physical fitness. The fascia participates in every movement—not just walking, dancing, and skipping, but also throwing and stretching.

Healthy fascia structures form protective joint capsules, contribute to core stability and a strong back, and are responsible for the body's muscle definition and contour. As a sensory organ they facilitate smooth, elegant movement, and they have a determining influence on how good and at home we feel in our bodies. So after years of neglect, there are plenty of reasons to pay more attention to this fascinating network.

Healthy fascia: Harmonic movement

Our body consists of a surprisingly large portion of fascia. In an adult this amounts to about 39 to 51 lbs of connective tissue that, depending on composition and structure, handles different tasks. To understand how tight and strong connective tissue is constructed we will take a closer look at the fascia of skeletal muscles. They participate in every movement, allow us to stand upright or sit, to walk and run. But they also participate when we twist, squirm, and squat, when we move our head or throw a ball. The reason is that the skeletal muscles are surrounded and permeated by a network of fascia arranged according to a smart biological blueprint.

Fascia: The Whole-Body Network

The muscular connective tissue is a three-dimensional mesh that permeates the body in every possible direction: from top to bottom, from front to back, from the outside to the inside. As the name connective tissue aptly suggests, as a whole-body network it weaves structures together. Depending on function and load, it forms high-tensile bands and coarse membranes, but also very flexible sheaths and delicate sacs.

The muscular connective tissue essentially consists of collagen fibers and connective tissue cells as well as lots of water. The collagen fibers compress into flat membranes according to body context and demand, but they also weave together in seemingly endless continuity into the innermost part of the muscle. Intramuscular collagen looks like delicate gossamer that continues to unravel to enmesh every single muscle fiber. That is why in this book we repeatedly refer to the collagen network.

The orange model

We like to use the orange model to gain a better understanding of how fascia is organized within the body. When you remove the orange peel and look at it from the inside, the white fibrous tissue is like the surface fascia (fascia superficialis), the subcutaneous fatty tissue. This upper layer is clearly separate from the next subjacent one because you are holding the peel in one hand and, separately, the enveloped flesh of the fruit as a compact whole in the other hand.

Analogously, underneath its subcutaneous fat tissue the human body has muscle fiber that is completely enveloped by the immediately subjacent deep fascia (fascia profunda).

In class I call this layer the catsuit, because it should ideally hold us together like a tight-fitting leotard. This layer is permeated by lots of nerves and blood vessels, and in our youth possesses considerable tension—at least as long as the collagen fibers are tight and toned. As we get older, the collagen fibers inevitably come apart at the seams due to lack of exercise or poor lifestyle choices. The body then loses tonicity, becomes flaccid, and we lose our previous well-defined body shape.

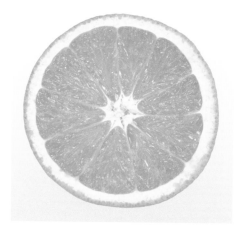

Striking similarity: Whether orange or human, both consist of lots of water neatly packaged via the bag-in-bag principle.

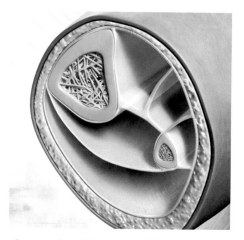

Cross-section of the human thigh: Connective tissue structures the body into so-called septa, similar to orange segments.

Of sections and septa

Let's stick with the orange model. Next, we separate the fruit into individual segments. Inside the muscle the fascia forms separating walls called septa. They subdivide the muscle into smaller functional units. Similar to orange segments, individual muscles are also packaged inside a collagen sheath, the so-called epimysium. If you open up an orange segment, the juice runs out, but when you take a closer look you can see that the sweet liquid is packaged in more delicate sacs. Transferring this to the organization inside the muscle, these correspond to the intramuscular connective tissue, the perimysium. But the continuity of our collagen network goes even farther. As a microstructure, it enmeshes every individual muscle fiber. This ultra-thin connective-tissue layer is called endomysium.

According to Robert Schleip, PhD, "our skeletal muscles usually don't consist of a single cord that is attached to the bone. If that were the case, they would not be as flexible and simultaneously strong and tear-resistant to be able to perform all kinds of movements." This means that, based on a specific building principle, our muscles are made of thousands of fibers that feed into a particularly resistant fascial tissue, the tendons, and after that adhere to the periosteum, or rather certain insertions on the bone. In nature, the sheath-to-sheath principle has proven effective for the structure of skeletal muscles, where multiple muscle fibers are bundled inside individual sheaths, and an outer sheath again envelops multiple muscle bundles.

If you look at a muscle from the inside to the outside you can see three types of sheaths:

1. Endomysium (endo = inside, within): These ultra-thin fascia surrounds every muscle fiber.

2. Perimysium (peri = around, surrounding): These fascial sheaths bundle together multiple muscle fibers that are covered by the endomysium. Since these bundles rest next to each other in a tube, they form the separating walls within.

3. Epimysium (epi = on, across, upon): This is the outer fascia sheath that surrounds the entire muscle and holds together all of the muscle fiber bundles in a sort of tube. The epimysium consists of connective tissue that is ideally one half to one millimeter thick.

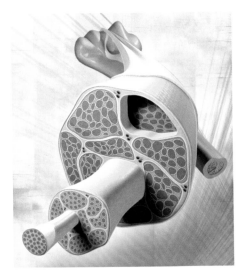

A whole-body network envelopes, permeates, and interweaves all muscles. In doing so, the protein component collagen weaves itself into a flexible sheath around the muscle, divides into more delicate sacs surrounding individual muscle bundles, then interweaves these in the form of fine gossamer within the muscle, and finally enmeshes each individual muscle fiber.

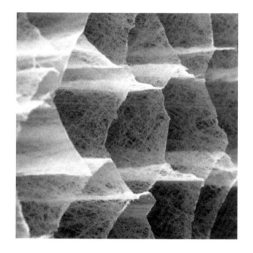

The finest fibers: This image shows the fine sheath surrounding individual muscle fibers, the endomysium. Impressive is the geometric bio structure reminiscent of honeycomb.

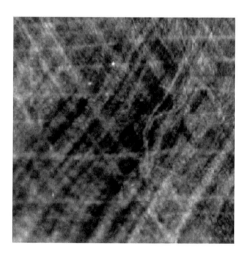

This orderly lattice structure is characteristic of young and healthy fascia. Anatomy professor Carla Stecco (Padua University) discovered that the angle is exactly 78 degrees. This lattice structure can be found in the muscle sheaths and the epimysium.

An adaptable network

During fascia training, we utilize the anatomy of continuity and are impressed by the collagen tissue's enormous adaptability. Resilient membranes or traction-resistant chords (but also flexible sheaths) form according to physical demand and context.

For example, if you touch the outside of your thigh it usually feels more defined and firm than the inside. The outside of a toddler's thigh is still just as soft as the inside. Because we respond to the challenge to stand up and walk on two legs, we evolve into a kind of "long-legged human animal" with ability to run, walk, and skip, fostering a strong, elastic, and force-resistant membrane on the outside of our thigh. But like with muscle and bones, if you don't use it, you lose it. In walking and running we naturally put strain on the soft tissue. They will respond with creating more sturdy, collagen-filled fibers. The opposite is true for an notorious coach potato and the associated lack of movement and loading. The formerly tight and toned fascial membrane loses firmness and structure. On top of that, we sacrifice inherent capacities gained from evolution and biology over millions of years, such as a light-footed, smooth gait or the highly efficient long-distance running. Add to that the loss of aesthetics because all of this makes the thighs flaccid and shapeless.

But the ability to shape tissue is also an incentive. Over time, adequate training stimulus can make collagen structures strong and firm again. That is why our motivating motto is: Train your fascia, tone your body!

The body as a river

With all the excitement about the versatility of collagen fibers, we must not forget one thing: Connective tissue consists of fibers, but mostly—like an orange—it consists of fluid. By the same token you could also say that the largest volume share in tissue is water and it was skillfully packaged inside the human organism based on the bag-in-bag principle as a clever evolutionary invention. It is still a largely unappreciated fact that the living body consists mostly of the saline primordial ocean from which our ancestors emerged half a billion years ago. That means modern humans are also cleverly packaged water (with 50 to 70% water content, depending on age) that nature has integrated into a collagen network of countless sacs and bags. The findings from modern water research are of great importance to fascia training and its fluid dynamics. You can read more on this topic in chapter 3.

A Tight Skin Is More Important Than Lots of Filler

At this point, I would like to introduce the sausage skin and sausage filler model. A sausage consists of a doughy mass that is contained by the skin. This metaphor is easy to understand because muscle mass is packed into the fascia sheath surrounding the muscle, the epimysium.

In order to have a toned body contour, it is not necessary to build up lots of mass and walk around like a pumped-up Michelin Man (provided that's not your beauty ideal). If the surrounding collagen sheath is strong and toned, lean muscles will have a clearly defined and graceful shape. Even if a body has a higher percentage of fat, the body shape is rounder and softer and has a more feminine shape thanks to toned and youthful fascia.

Only when collagen begins to slacken does the subcutaneous fat begin to look flabby and the previously round and feminine shape goes to seed. So being slender isn't just about muscle mass and percentage of body fat, but also about the tension of the enveloping connective tissue (i.e., the fascia).

During a laboratory visit, I found out why that is important: The researchers placed a slice of firm flesh in a test tube and added an enzyme that preserves the red muscle fibers and within a few hours only dissolves the whitish collagen fibers. After that the flesh had lost its previously firm consistency and behaved similar to thick syrup when the test tube was tilted.

When applying this to fascia training, it tells us that we must focus on specifically tightening the intramuscular connective tissue. On the other hand, the sheath around the muscle must also be strengthened and tightened. That is why we have developed new exercises in collaboration with Robert Schleip, PhD, and his colleagues. They are intended to stimulate connective tissue cells, the fibroblasts, in the collagen network of the muscle sheath to generate more fibers. This principle is based on the motto "It's more about the skin and less about the sausage."

To understand this effective training principle, it is necessary to get better acquainted with the fibroblasts and the connective tissue cells as the architect.

At a glance
The 7 most important fascia chains

Upper-body fascia
1. Shoulder-elbow chain
2. Chest-biceps chain

Core fascia
3. Abdominal network: straight, oblique, and transverse abdominal muscles

Back fascia
4. Diagonal lat-glutes muscle chain

Lower-body fascia
5. Plantar fascia-heel pad-Achilles tendon chain
6. Foot arch-adductors-pelvic floor chain
7. Fascia lata: the fascia of the thigh

The 7 Most Important Fascia Chains

The fascia interpenetrates our entire body and interlinks as so-called myofascial chains. Tom Myers, who gave an impressive description of the myofascial lines of pull, previously brought this anatomical principle of interconnected tension to light. We will introduce the most important fascia lines below. In the practical part of the book, you will find specific exercises for each chain that will create a full-body fascia-toning workout.

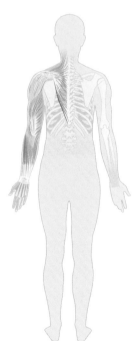

1. Shoulder-elbow chain

This chain runs from the outside of the forearm to the elbow and on to the outside of the upper arm with the important lateral septum that connects to the deltoid muscle fascia (Musculus deltoideus), which extends from the upper part of the trapezius muscle (Musculus trapezius) to the neck. It also extends from the middle and lower part of the trapezius muscle to the spine.

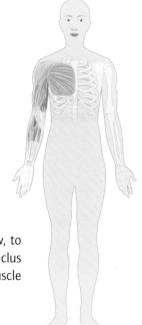

2. Chest-biceps chain

This line runs from the inside of the forearm, via the elbow, to the flexor side of the upper arm, including the biceps (Musuclus biceps brachii). It then connects to the large pectoral muscle (Musculus pectoralis major) all the way to the sternum.

3. The abdominal network: straight, oblique, and transverse

The abdominal network is multi-layer and runs in multiple directions: straight, oblique, and transverse. This meshwork extends to the transverse abdominal muscle (Musculus transversus abdominus), which connects to the pelvic floor.

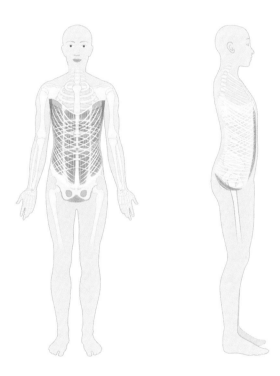

The straight abdominal muscle (Musculus rectus abdominus) forms the uppermost, vertical layer, running from the pubis to the sternum. The second, deeper layer runs diagonally and is formed by the external oblique muscle (Musculus obliquus externus abdominis), which runs along the side of the ribcage from the top outside to the bottom. From there it weaves its meshes further into the internal oblique muscle (Musculus obliquus internus abdominus), which runs downward and to the outside. Beneath that is the transverse abdominal muscle that, together with the pelvic floor, forms the innermost layer. This deep transverse layer also forms an internal fascial corset that extends all the way around the deepest layer of the thoracolumbar fascia (Fascia thoracolumbalis) and thereby also stabilizes the lumbar vertebra.

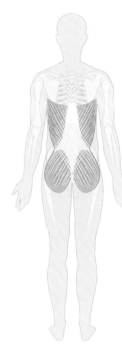

4. Diagonal lat-glutes muscle chain

This ample diagonal line spans from the large gluteal muscle (Musculus glutaeus maximus) to the large back muscle (Musculus latissimus dorsi) and is covered by the thoracolumbar fascia's superficial layer. It connects the upper body to the lower body and this chain's elasticity influences the swinging of arms and legs as we walk, among other things. Because the thoracolumbar fascia forms a dense connective tissue membrane, we can assume that this means a healthy back is capable of taking heavy loads and high impacts. Plus, strong tissues and well-toned fascia sheaths around the glutes are the best guarantee for a tight butt.

5. Plantar fascia-heel pad-Achilles tendon chain

This chain is formed by the fibrous covering along the bottom of the foot. It extends from the fleshy part of the toes to the heel and is called the plantar fascia (Aponeurosis plantaris). The plantar fascia compacts toward the heel pad that covers the heel bone. The pad can shift easily and connects to the posterior part of the Achilles tendon, which has a longer extension, the Achilles aponeurosis, that reaches to the knee.

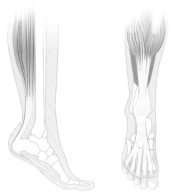

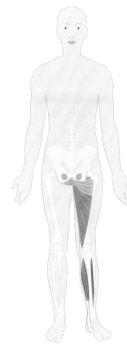

6. Foot arch-adductors-pelvic floor chain

This chain extends from the inside of the foot between heel and inner malleolus to the inside of the lower leg. It runs deep inside the lower leg between the tibia and fibula in front of the calf muscles and from there to the inside of the knee. This fascia strengthens the knee joint capsule as well as the knee ligaments. This chain continues on to the adductor group, a compact muscle group at the inside of the thigh. The adductors (Musculus adductor magnus, Musculus adductor longus, Musculus adductor brevis, Musculus adductor minimus, Musculus gracilis and Musculus pectineus) insert into the pelvis and connect into the anterior portion of the pelvic floor.

7. Fascia lata: the fascia of the thigh

This large fascia begins at the iliac crest and from here runs along the outside of the thigh to just below the knee. The large gluteal muscle and the tensor fascia latae—a small but strong muscle that originates at the anterior pelvic brim—work together as membrane tighteners. In training, we award this magical seventh fascia special status for tightening connective tissue because the thigh fascia and its special shape at the outside of the thigh, the Tractus iliotibialis, are responsible for a toned contour. This fascia therefore plays a central role when it comes to cellulite and in chapter 5 we devote some special thigh-shaping exercises

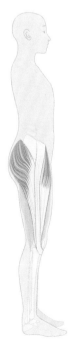

Ingenious Tissue Architecture

Studies show that collagen tissue in young people as well as well-trained myofascial tissues often have a lattice-like structure. This applies specifically to tissue that is stretched in different directions on a daily basis. Ideally the muscle is not only stretch loaded in length like a tendon, but also widthwise, which is the case when the muscle

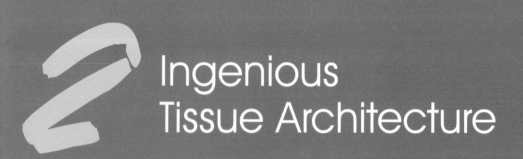

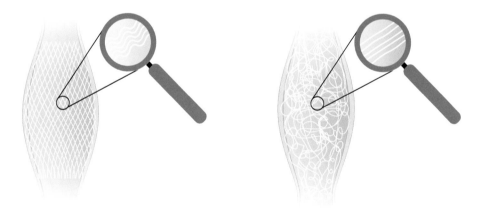

If you don't move, you get rusty. With lack of exercise, the fascia loses its lattice-like alignment, sprawls in every direction, and literally becomes matted. In addition, the wavy microstructure of individual collagen fibers is lost and with it the springy, elastic tension (image on the right).

fibers contract, creating bulky belly muscle. The lattice-like architecture of the fibers handles these different demands ingeniously. The following illustration shows how these structures change in the course of our lives if we don't get enough exercise.

Connective tissue: the movement organ

"You have got to move!" This demand applies particularly to the fascia. This apt assertion comes from the renowned sports physician and doctor for the German national soccer team, Dr. Müller-Wohlfahrt, who some years ago published a book with that title on the athletic trainability of connective tissue.

When connective tissue is young and elastic, the microstructure of the individual collagen fibers is clearly corrugated. Scientists assume that this cunning construction plan is an essential basis for the elastic storage capacity of well-trained collagen. This phenomenal ability to store kinetic energy short term and then vigorously release it enables happy skipping, bouncing, or an efficient running performance.

As it ages, but most of all from lack of exercise, the tissue loses its lattice-like macro- and wave-like microstructure. The collagen fibers no longer react to tensile stress like an elastic spring, but rather more like a brittle rope. The fibers sprawl wildly in every direction, form lots of crosslinks, and get matted. Everyday movements become awkward and labored. We are no longer able to bend over as easily to, for instance, tie our shoes or we lose that springy tension when we climb stairs. This is caused not only by the weak, shortened muscles but more especially by the fascia fibers that have become brittle.

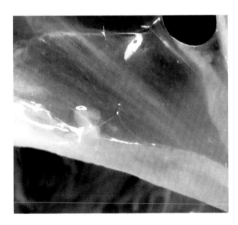

A healthy fascia is juicy. The youthfulness and slipperiness of collagen tissue is largely determined by the dynamics of the liquid matrix.

Myofibroblasts: Collagen Tissue Architects

Five questions to Robert Schleip, PhD

A healthy body immediately reacts to injuries to the outside of the skin or to the inside that are caused by an accident or an operation. The local tissue sends signals as quickly as possible to trigger multiple cell reactions one-by-one with the goal of closing the wound with a scar.

1. Which cells are particularly active during the healing process?

   Schleip, PhD: "They are the myofibroblasts that we have done quite a bit of research on at Ulm University. I call them supermen because they are four times as strong and produce much more collagen than the ordinary fibroblasts from which they originated."

2. What is the function of fibroblasts?

   Schleip, PhD: "Fibroblasts are ordinary jack-of-all-trades cells in the connective tissue. For instance, they produce collagen, but they also eat it when it gets old. They perform this task with most of the other components of the matrix that surrounds them."

3. And what happens with a fresh wound?

   Schleip, PhD: "Many fibroblasts transform themselves within a few days after an injury. Previously they functioned like Clark Kent, whom we know as the ordinary guy from comics and movies, and who just goes about his usual job.

But when an injury causes the fibroblasts to enter a certain biochemical and mechanical environment they, within a few hours to a few days, develop into particularly active myofibroblasts and, much like Clark Kent, suddenly turn into Superman."

4. During the initial phase of an injury, the myofibroblasts produce particularly more collagen, which speeds up the healing process and greatly contracts the surrounding fiber network in order to close the wound. What happens during the second phase?

Schleip, PhD: "A healthy, normal myofibroblast continues to behave like a superman only when it makes sense to do so. So if he has closed the wound and the tissue is strong enough to withstand stresses and strains, he commits a kind of honorable suicide and disappears. Doctors refer to this type of seppuku as apoptosis."

5. Once a wound has healed and their work is done, the myofibroblasts disappear. But as we know from Superman, myofibroblasts also have weaknesses. So why is it that they can cause problems during the second phase of wound repair?

Schleip, PhD: "One disadvantage of myofibroblasts is that while they can produce lots of collagen, they are less good at removing their own waste later on. This results in a thickening of the tissue at the edge of the wound, called fibrosis. It is the remaining, visible scar. This happens particularly with myofibroblasts that, for whatever reason, refuse to make way for other more useful tissue elements via apoptosis after their work is done."

Fibrosis

The term *fibrosis* refers to oathological connective tissue growths. They can develop as part of wound repair or for other reasons, such as overloading, which is often the case with professional athletes. But the most common cause of fibrosis, meaning the loss of the orderly lattice-like architecture of the fibers, is the underloading of tissue from a pervasive lack of movement and exercise. Characteristics are chaotic proliferation of fibers, matting, and adherance to other structures. In short, the fascia becomes brittle.

If you don't move, you get sticky

Nature designed the human body so the dense membranous fascia sheets are connected via loose connective tissue. You can visualize these natural adhesions as small spider webs that form loose connective tissue, filling the spaces between neighboring dense fascia layers. They facilitate smooth movements but don't allow complete free gliding.

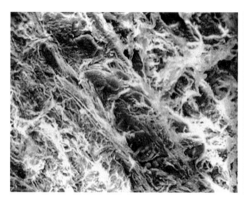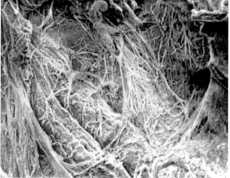

Fluffy fibers as shown in the image on the left, are a sign of healthy collagen. By contrast, the fibers on the right are brittle, frequently caused by lack of exercise.

But what happens when the fascia is too closely connected to the muscle sheaths beneath (i.e., adhering to them)? Researchers have been able to show in several studies that in many people with chronic back pain the thoracolumbar fascia adheres much too closely to the underlying muscle sheath. They now speculate that lots of chronic soft tissue pain, particularly in the back, is linked to poorly gliding flat fascia.

Robert Schleip, PhD, estimates that "80 percent of all back operations are unnecessary." The fascia researcher therefore recommends getting a second opinion from another physician or expert to also have the connective tissue more closely examined via ultrasound. If the fascia is locally thickened and sticky, Schleip recommends targeted and regular fascia training. There is a good chance that you will be able to move pain-free again after a few weeks or months.

Stress Promotes Hardening of the Fascia

The daily madness we usually refer to as stress, and which is accompanied by constant agitation and a lack of regeneration and balance in the autonomic nervous system, also affects the fascia network. The immediacy with which the nervous system and stress affect the fascia surprised even the researchers.

Under the influence of specific transmitters, the fibroblasts increase their activity, producing more collagen fibers and wiring the fibers particularly tight together. The stress-sensitive trapezoid muscle in the upper shoulder area then feels like it has been washed and shrunken in hot water. We call this tension; on the collagen level it is called a contracture. The problem is that this hardening persists even after the connective tissue cells have stopped their overzealous activity. Releasing the contracture can then require special measures to unmat the collagen over time and let it become smooth again. The expert hands of a myofascial therapist, working with a foam roller, and melting stretches are helpful here.

The Two Sides of Fascial Viscoelasticity

Floppy or toned—is it all a question of time? Or does our genetic predisposition play a role here? It is a valid question because we carry with us a basic genetic collagen structure, and this genetic component determines the appearance of cellulite, among other things (see page 151).

Our genes help to determine whether we tend toward a flexible, elastic, or a rather sturdy but stiff connective tissue type.

This question of type depends on another one of collagen's characteristics because the versatile protein fiber is characterized by a combination of two different properties: viscosity and elasticity.

Viscosity

Honey is a viscous fluid and in spite of its softness it resists the spoon that stirs it. This is called viscosity. In collagen tissues, this property of viscosity is responsible for the pliability and flexibility of the fibers. Depending on the type, they can be more soft on one side and tend to wear out during loading. This is true with a long run as well as the well-known phenomenon, the classic forward bend: If at the beginning of the exercise the fingertips are still a couple of inches from the floor, they gradually move closer to the floor or even touch it when the increased position is held for 30-60 seconds. In Hatha yoga this is a desired effect to temporarily increase flexibility. This form of stretching (i.e., holding a position and relaxing into it) is called melting stretches.

But in the following minutes to hours these tissues contract back to their original length. This creep effect comes with an associated energy loss; the elasticity and resilience of collagen fibers is temporarily lowered. It is therefore not recommended to do melting stretches right before an athletic competition or dynamic movements.

Elasticity

Elasticity refers to resilient strength, particularly in tissues that are subjected to dynamic forces. The fibrous band at the sole of the foot is a good example. If our plantar fascia was as flexible as gelatin, we would not be able to walk any faster than a sloth.

The strong collagen membranes or tendons have a high storage capacity. Similar to an elastic spring, they can absorb kinetic energy and release it again without any appreciable loss.

How elasticity functions has been impressively documented via ultrasound tests on the human Achilles tendon. It lengthens maximally right before takeoff—similar to a tight rubber band—and in doing so it stores energy and then releases it during the jump.

Conclusion: Healthy fascia is elastic, resilient, and springy. Yet it must be trained through adequate loading stimuli.

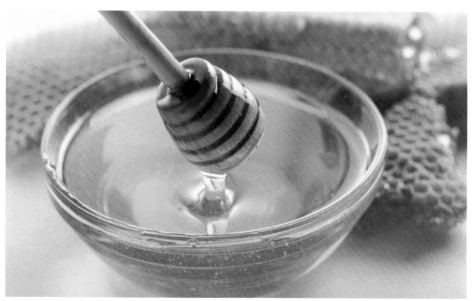

Collagen is viscoelastic, which refers to two outstanding properties of the protein fibers that are omnipresent in the human body: elastic like a steel spring and viscous like honey.

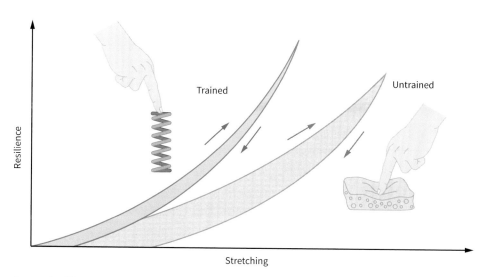

Sport scientific research has shown that tissue that was previously soft like a saggy mattress can be reshaped within weeks and months to elastic spring-like properties via targeted fascia training.

Evolutionary Biology

What do top model Eva Padberg, musician Lady Gaga, and actors Angelina Jolie and Brad Pitt have in common? They swear by yoga and for years have been practicing poses that seem to be unachievable by the average person.

Even if you are not a yoga fan, surely you have asked yourself why it is that some people are born to do yoga. This extremely flexible species can bend their spines like serpents and their hip joints don't seem to be subject to earthly laws when it comes to contortions. These people usually move through life with the elegant grace of temple dancers, and from head to toe match the pervasive slender-beautiful-supple criteria of the staunch yoga community. Good karma?

Other serious yoga disciples labor for years and do not nearly achieve this graceful flexibility. In extreme cases, this inflexible type appears like a compact Viking who mistakenly ended up in a yoga class. He feels terrible and looks it, too. Bad karma?

You may find comfort in the fact that this is neither a case of personal deficiency nor just punishment for misdeeds in a former life. But it stands to reason that it is the properties of the muscular connective tissue that cause these significant differences in flexibility and mobility. Sometimes it is simply our genetic collagen configuration that decides whether we belong to the temple dancer group or the rather sturdy and stiff Viking types.

About the pendant earlobe and the loose tongue

Often you can even see externally whether or not you have soft and easily stretchy fascia. Take a look in the mirror. What does your earlobe look like? What kind of attachment do you see under your tongue? If you are a temple dancer type, you likely don't have attached earlobes but rather free-hanging ones. The reason: Soft connective tissue forms fewer crosslinks because the fibroblasts form only a few spider webs with which they can build bridges between tissues. Without sufficient crosslinks, the earlobes don't attach during embryonic development but rather form a pendant.

The same principle applies to the tongue frenulum. Try to roll your tongue all the way back. If it works, you have a thin, flexible tongue frenulum that only loosely connects tongue and palate. This would be an indication of the temple dancer type. If you are unable to roll up your tongue, the connective tissue in that location has become strongly fixed and connects tongue and palate close together.

To become better acquainted with these extreme forms we invite you to a scavenger hunt into the still largely unknown world of the fascia. First we will focus on the genetic causes of the two connective tissue types. And we will answer the following question: How did cold and heat affect the connective tissue structure in the course of evolution?

Women: the flexible gender?

Whether yoga, ballet, or gymnastics, it's usually girls and women who naturally tend to be hyperflexible and able to develop their flexibility further so they can demonstrate extreme body positions with ease. This includes, for instance, landing in a split from a jump or performing several backflips in a row.

Since women are considered potential mothers from a biological point of view, nature has made sure they are equipped with flexible connective tissue. It provides plenty of cushioning for the internal organs in the abdomen and the uterine tissue can expand during pregnancy to provide sufficient room for the baby.

But some men can also be surprisingly flexible. "Although girls and women are more often hyperflexible types than boys and men, there are also male contortionists who are able to extremely hyperextend their joints due to soft connective tissue," says Robert Schleip, PhD.

When we watch men in the circus and on the dance floor and in athletic gymnastics, who are flexible and move gracefully, we tend to be astonished. Probably also because our circle of friends and acquaintances seems to largely consist of inflexible men, the Viking types. Whether man or woman, Viking or temple dancer, whining doesn't work! Since your parents gave you that connective tissue type for life, you must make the best of it and engage in regular fascia training. In the practice portion of the book starting in chapter 5, you will learn which fascia training exercises are suitable to specifically strengthen and tighten the connective tissue.

Men with soft connective tissue: advantages and disadvantages

As far back as the fourth century BC, Hippocrates mentioned that there are people with a "flaccid physique." The most famous physician of antiquity also attributed these characteristics to the Scythians.

His assumption was that the flaccid nomadic horsemen lost so many battles because their shoulder and elbow joints weren't stable enough to properly draw a bow. But hypermobility of the joints along with soft connective tissue doesn't have to be an inherent physical disadvantage, as the example of the 18th century violinist Niccolò Paganini shows. The virtuoso is said to have played the notes so breathtakingly fast because he had such extremely flexible hands and fingers.

The (hyper)flexible temple dancers

When you were a child, did you ever try to do the splits in PE class? How well did you do? And if you succeeded, are you still able to do it today?

Whether or not you succeeded, many of us cannot remotely approach the level of extreme flexibility of some temple dancers and acrobats that perform in the ballet, circus, or variety shows. These people, whose graceful movements in yoga, ballet, or figure skating we admire, are genetically predisposed to having exceptionally flexible connective tissue. But every biological advantage also comes with a disadvantage. That often jealously admired flexibility exists at the expense of the tissue's sturdiness. Such soft and flexible connective tissue fails more easily under stress and strain than a sturdy, more resilient one.

Bones, joints, and vertebrae no longer have that springy cushioning that separates them. Collapsing on to each other, they wear down over the years. According to a comment by one of my class participant's orthopedic surgeon when he recently recommended she have a hip replacement: "Sooner or later all hyperflexible people get their turn."

But it doesn't have to be that way. According to Robert Schleip, PhD: "People of the average temple dancer type should not extensively stretch their collagen tissue, but rather do targeted strengthening. An additional benefit: outer sheath surrounding the muscles, the epimysium, will be tighter and the body contour will be better defined."

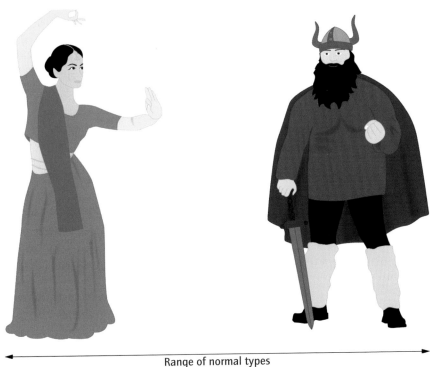

Range of normal types

Born to do yoga? Or are you a rather stiff but stable Viking? This is determined by the connective tissue's genetic configuration. Each type possesses functional advantages but also disadvantages.

Biological advantages of the temple dancer type

The temple dancer type's genetic configuration determines which biological advantages result. These people are able to move through difficult terrain over long distances, and are nimble climbers and light-footed runners. A high degree of flexibility is certainly an advantage for meeting the demands of a tropical jungle, a natural agility course with low-hanging branches, impassable obstacles, and high-hanging fruit.

Why did nature arrange it so people are born as temple dancer types? According to Schleip, PhD: "To date there are only hypotheses that are very plausible, particularly since they are based on results from previous studies. Researchers from the Netherlands have developed a theory I find reasonable. It states: Certain attributes were useful to our ancestors who survived well around a tropical steppe. And those were, among others, longer tendons and greater flexibility overall."

Imagine the following scenario: In the tropical rainforest, these flexible primordial human beings were more adept at gathering food and faster when escaping from an enemy if they were able to move quickly and nimbly through the forest without too much muscular effort. Not only moving through the tropical jungle, but also running through the hot steppe would have been life threatening had they been as stiff as Vikings. Here it was important to be able to run long distances without quickly overheating and getting tired. A long and elastic Achilles tendon and its energy-storing capacity made this possible without great muscular exertion.

If you have a naturally flexible fascia, you are the beneficiary of this evolutionary legacy. You are able to move gracefully and use your limbs supply. You probably also have long Achilles tendons which, if they are well trained, might help you during endurance runs. As a mother-to-be, you have less trouble giving birth because the ligaments of your pelvis are long and flexible. You also won the lottery from a cosmetic point of view. Your wounds may heal more slowly, but afterwards your skin is smooth again. Robert Schleip, PhD: "Asian women, who are often temple dancer types, heal nearly without scars, and that even after many cosmetic surgeries."

Flexibility and the psyche

Statistics show that temple temple dancer types develop an anxious personality more often than people with a more robust build. Robert Schleip, PhD, surmises a correlation between motor function and psyche: "When hyperflexible children don't feel as physically sturdy during adolescence and struggle with heavy loads more than others do, that experience can mold their self-confidence. They may become more cautious and fearful when the next challenge or test of courage arises, but we should beware of the inference that all hyperflexible people are petulant and neurotic. That is most certainly false."

Biological disadvantages of the temple dancer type

Extremely flexible people often already show physical symptoms as children that can last into adulthood. Three quarters of those afflicted develop unspecific and chronic pain between the ages of 13 and 19, particularly girls. Often a first indicator is that children and adolescents demonstrate the feat of severely hyperextending their fingers and thumbs (see the test on page 42).

But when they spend many hours writing or do a lot of work on the computer, it can result in pain. Often the hip creaks during certain movements, but creaking joints can also affect fingers, the jaw, and the vertebrae. Joint pain and swelling most often occurs in the legs and feet, and instability of the lumbar spine can also lead to fascial pain. Robert Schleip, PhD, suspects that "growing pains above the knee are often associated with hypermobility." Most temple dancer types develop flat feet and sliding disks at some point in their lives, and they often suffer from back pain. These symptoms can intensify due to excess weight, sitting for hours on end, and too little physical exercise. It is also more likely that the vertebrae as well as the sacroiliac joint dislocate during everyday movements.

Additionally, very soft connective tissue isn't particularly robust and is therefore unable to keep bones well separated. The result is that in their youth temple dancer types often suffer from scoliosis. This causes the spine to curve laterally so bodyweight is distributed unevenly, which can be very painful.

Weak connective tissue does not handle strain very well so even a little pressure can result in contusions. It unfortunately also fails easily, which is why very pregnant women and newly delivered mothers often suffer from posterior pelvic pain and for weeks have problems when standing.

Women with supersoft connective tissue sooner or later develop dimples, dents, and bumps on their thighs, buttocks, stomach, and upper arms. Doctors refer to this type of orange-peel skin as cellulite, not to be confused with cellulitis, which indicates inflammation in the subcutaneous tissue. You can read about how cellulite develops via a complex interplay of fascial and hormonal changes on page 151.

Often overlooked: hypermobility and pain

Many temple dancer types suffer from pain because of their hypermobility. Doctors often misdiagnose back pain and suspect blockages or tension as the cause.

About Vikings
and Temple Dancers

Three questions to Robert Schleip, PhD

1. What does our ancestry have to do with whether or not we are naturally hypermobile?

    Schleip, PhD: "Studies on hypermobility show that there are three important influencing factors: gender, age, and ethnic origin. Hypermobility is therefore more prevalent in girls and women. Children are also more flexible, whereby this flexibility decreases with age. Particularly exciting for us fascia researchers is that hypermobility is particularly prevalent in people of south Asian and African descent.

    By contrast, people whose ancestors hail from northern Europe tend to develop particularly rigid connective tissue more so than others. That is good for stability but makes one less flexible. It also appears to promote a predisposition to the so-called Viking disease or Dupuytren's contracture that is particularly common in older men and is characterized by a shortening of the palmar fascia located in the palm.*

    We call people who constitutionally tend to a stiffening of the connective tissue Viking types. On a continuous spectrum, Viking types and temple dancer types are the two extremes."

2. What are the supporting numbers?

    Schleip, PhD: "I would estimate that there are more stiff Viking types than flexible dancer types in Germany. I deduce this from previous studies on the occurrence of hypermobility. They show that only 5 percent of adult Americans are hypermobile, compared to 25-30 percent of Iraqis, and as much as 43 percent of the Yoruba tribe in Nigeria.

In the course of evolution the fascial variation that contains softer and more flexible connective tissue appears to have established itself more successfully in tropical climate zones than in arctic ones. It is therefore no coincidence that yoga developed in India where, with the exception of the mountain regions, there is a subtropical climate with temperatures as warm as 122° F."

3.   And who is in the middle on the mobility scale?

Schleip, PhD: "Since the scale is a continuum there exists many mixed types. These crossover types can check additional characteristics of the temple dancer type by taking the flexibility test. If multiple criteria coincide, the mixed types move from their position in the middle closer to the temple dancer type. **

But the muscular connective tissue is not only affected by genetic configuration but also by lifestyle. The demands you place on your body don't make an award-winning temple dancer out of a ready-for-Hollywood Viking, or vice-versa, but it can absolutely lead to individual local areas shifting toward stiffening or toward flexibility. Then the fascia of muscles that is frequently condemned to long-term static effort tends to stiffen while chronically under-challenged muscles tend to atrophy. For instance, the myofascial tissue at the neck is often stiff, which is also associated with the very common forward head posture in daily life."

*   You can read more about the health problems of hypermobile people on page 36.

**   You can read more about the additional characteristics of hypermobility in the test on page 42.

Conclusion on Fascia Training

Now you probably have a better understanding of your own body and its peculiarities. As a temple dancer type, enjoy the natural gifts of flexibility, elegance, and grace. But you also have a little more trouble with stability than a classic Viking type does. Try to carry a child on your shoulders. You will likely get tired quickly and at least temporarily wish for the more robust build of an Obelix-like Viking.

For an all-around sense of well-being, joint health, and also a toned instead of a floppy body shape, you should purposefully strengthen your connective tissue. Extensive stretching, even if it is one of your favorite activities, is only of limited benefit to you. To create healthy and strong connective tissue, you must tone your fascia tissue and build more muscle tone in the weeks and months ahead. Start your training with the exercises on page 105.

The Czech muscle researcher Vladimir Janda (1927-2002) already described muscular imbalance patterns that are particularly common in Western industrialized nations. They distinguish body types that correspond to the rather more flexible and flaccid tissue type of the temple dancer, but in other areas of the body are stiff and tight like a Viking. The illustration on page 44, which depicts the typical imbalances of the crossover type, shows a slightly modified progression of these imbalanced patterns. Take the corresponding self-test to find out easily how this crossover pattern applies to you and which areas of the body you need to strengthen accordingly.

Are you curious now? In the practical part of the book, beginning in chapter 5, we will introduce the appropriate strength exercises for each fascia chain.

The Temple Dancer Test and Crossover Test

Four questions to Robert Schleip, PhD

1. Why should we find out if we are a temple dancer type or a crossover type?

    Robert Schleip, PhD: "The two self-tests are useful for identifying initial information. When you figure out that you are more one type or the other, you will have a better understanding of your body. During the next step, you can then train your connective tissue individually, purposefully strengthen it where the structure is too soft and flaccid, and create more flexibility in those areas that are too stiff and rigid. If you have serious problems with some of the exercises, you should consult a trusted physician for a thorough examination of your tissue and joints."

2. What do the two tests screen for?

    Robert Schleip, PhD: "They are flexibility tests. During the first self-test, you will do exercises that will indicate a constitutional tendency toward elastic and flexible connective tissue (i.e., the flexible temple dancer type). During the second test, you will check to see if you would benefit from tightening the muscular connective tissue, in a few specific areas rather than the entire body. That would make you more of a crossover type.

    The basic idea is to find movements for this test that are representative and encompass a significant distinction. It isn't just about that one joint you move the most during an exercise. Usually several joints and the surrounding tissue are involved."

3. How was the temple dancer test created?

Robert Schleip, PhD: "There were multiple precursors and studies until the researchers agreed on the final form. In recent years, the temple dancer test, known as the Beighton Test in professional circles, has been validated as both sensitive and convincing."

4. Why should some people follow up with a second test?

Robert Schleip, PhD: "If you find, after taking the first test, that you have very few characteristics of a flexible temple dancer type, you may be more of a crossover type.

You then take the second test to find out where you are on the spectrum. As you do so, you figure out which parts of your body are not flexible. Of course it is possible that you are neither a temple dancer type nor a crossover type. But you can still benefit from the following practical exercises to tighten connective tissue if, for instance, you do them for esthetic reasons, to maintain or give the body a better shape."

Test: Are You a Temple Dancer Type?

To find out if you are a temple dancer type and would therefore benefit from strengthening your connective tissue, get into the positions shown in the illustrations in consecutive order. Give yourself a Yes point if your position resembles the one in the book. Your maximum score for each individual test is one point.

Forward bend test:

Can you touch the floor with your palms when you bend forward with your knees fully extended?

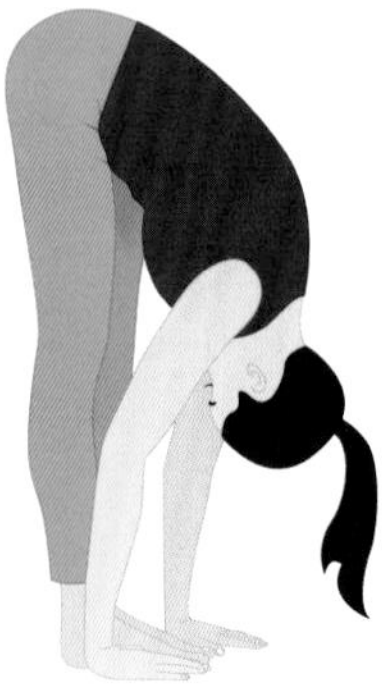

Points

Elbow hyperextension:

Are you able to hyperextend your elbow by 10 degrees or more?

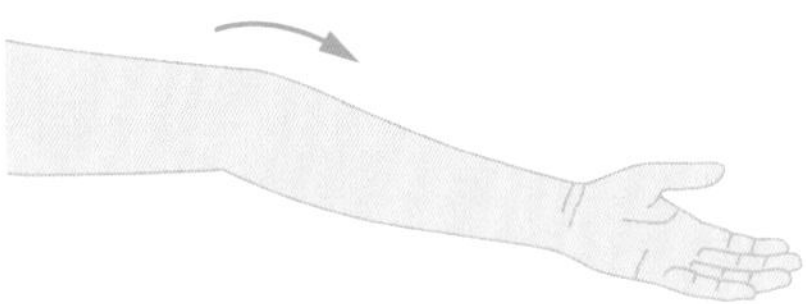

Right

Left

Knee hyperextension

Are you able to hyperextend your knee by 10 degrees or more?

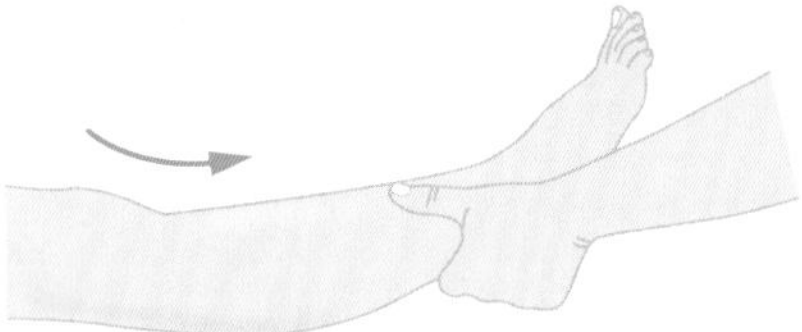

Right

Left

		Points
Thumb-to-forearm test:		
Are you able to rest your thumb against your forearm?		
	Right	
	Left	
Finger hyperextension:		
Are you able to hyperextend your pinkie by 90 degrees or more?		
	Right	
	Left	
Total points (9 points max.)		

Score

6 or more points:

You are most likely a very flexible person of the temple dancer type with rather more soft and flexible connective tissue.

4 to 5 points:

Based solely on this test, your classification is not conclusive. A genetic predisposition to softer connective tissue is likely if several of the following characteristics apply:

- Pendant earlobes
- Thin and flexible tongue frenulum
- Propensity to contusions in daily life

- Developed scoliosis during puberty

- Slow or delayed wound healing

- Propensity to joint dislocation in daily life

1 to 3 points:

You have no genetic predisposition to general hypermobility.

Test: Are You a Crossover Type?

The following flexibility tests will help you narrow down the areas in which you could most benefit from strengthening your connective tissue. If you have typical imbalances, it is an indication that you may be a crossover type. A fascial dysfunction indicates an imbalance. Some fascial elements are shortened, restricting their movement, while other fascial elements are weakened and should therefore be strengthened via training.

The following set of tests focuses on restricted mobility in specific areas. Give yourself two points each time the described restriction of range of motion definitely applies to you. Give yourself one point if the restriction somewhat applies to you. You get no points if you cannot detect a restriction of your range of motion.

	Points
Chin-to-chest test: While standing, tilt your head forward with your mouth closed and try to touch your chin to your sternum. If you have gone as far as you can and can still fit two or more fingers between your chin and your sternum, give yourself 2 points.	
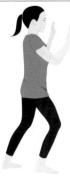 Knee-to-the-wall test: Stand facing a wall and place your palms against the wall at shoulder level. Push one foot forward until your toe touches the wall and bend your knee until it also touches the wall. Repeat by incrementally moving your foot ½ to 1 inch further away from the wall. Give yourself two points if you are unable to move either foot more than a hand-width away from the wall without your knee losing contact with the wall.	

	Points
Reclined angel test: Lie on your back and bend both elbows at a right angle. Elbows and upper arms rest on the floor at shoulder level. Without changing the elbow angle, slide your arms up overhead as far as you can without the elbows lifting off the floor. Give yourself two points if one upper arm can get closer to your head than 45 degrees.	
Hip extension test: In a prone position raise one leg with the knee bent while placing one hand on your low back to feel for a definite increase in the arch in your back. Give yourself two points if you are unable to lift either knee more than a hand's length off the floor without arching your back.	
Total points (8 points max.)	

Score

6 to 8 points:
Your test results show definite signs of typical crossover imbalances.

3 to 5 points:
There is tendential evidence, but these test results alone are not conclusive.

0 to 2 points:
You are not a typical crossover type.

If the test shows you to be a crossover type, you should do the exercises for tightening connective tissue, particularly those marked in purple in the illustration, and described in the practical part of the book.

However, for the areas marked in blue we recommend you follow the guidelines on page 95 for Viking types as well as individual regional Viking tissues.

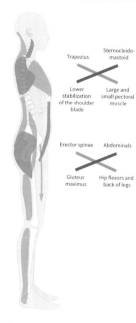

Trapezius
Sternocleido-mastoid
Lower stabilization of the shoulder blade
Large and small pectoral muscle
Erector spinae
Abdominals
Gluteus maximus
Hip flexors and back of legs

Areas that tend to shorten and misalign
Areas that tend to slacken

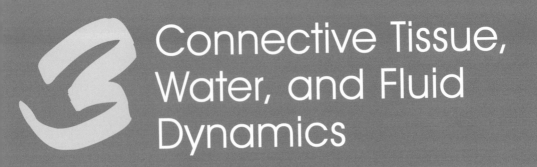

Connective Tissue, Water, and Fluid Dynamics

We look at our bodies as something solid, tangible, substantial. But we are seldom aware of the fact that our bodies are two-thirds water and we may not be as solidly built as we assume.

Water is an exceptional element. Its many anomalies make it the elixir of life and it controls life on our planet. Our individual evolution takes place in the primordial ocean of the uterus. Our collective human history originated billions of years ago, in the primordial ocean from which our ancestors emerged onto dry land.

As two-legged land dwellers, each of us carries a piece of primordial ocean around our planet for our whole lives. Even in modern times of smart phones and high-speed Internet, a piece of the ancient ocean lives within us. The salt and mineral content of today's oceans has changed over time, but the primordial ocean's composition still flows within our fluid system, and thus within the basic substance of our connective tissue.

The body as a fluid event

As Heraclitus so aptly said: "You could not step twice into the same rivers; for other waters are ever flowing onto you." This is also true for the living and healthy organism. Water's essence lies in its constant change and continuous transformation. On this level, the body is not a fixed entity, but rather flows like a river. Anyone taking a look at the impressive photos taken by the hand surgeon Jean-Claude Guimberteau will agree with this assertion. The French physician was the first to show connective tissue in vivo, meaning in a living human being. He takes us into the fascinating world of loose connective tissue with his endoscopic camera and calls his journey through the body "Promenades sous la peau," a walk under the skin. And what do we discover? A constantly changing and continuously reconfiguring gelatinous tissue continuum of impressive tensile strength. Three new branches form in quick succession while simultaneously two existing ones in another place dissolve. Moreover, we are astounded by the obvious moisture within these structures including subtly dispersed droplets that travel along the fibers, reminiscent of glistening dewdrops in a spider web.

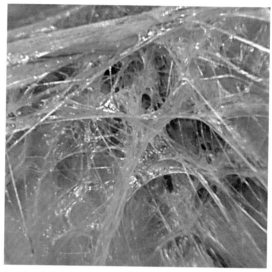

Fascinating fascia: This endoscopic image gives us a rare view of the superficial layer of connective tissue just below the skin of a living organism.

Misleading anatomy

Anatomically speaking, the difference between a living organism and a corpse could not be plainer: Anatomical specimens are lifeless bodies, meaning without movement, without feeling, without vitality. No wonder the anatomists of the past were misled and completely overlooked the body in its fluid reality. The mechanistic science of the past century and its conviction that the functions of a body can explained through fragmentation had to fail because of the body's fluid dynamics. A river cannot be dissected into individual parts; it has no countable fragments that can be added up.

Unfortunately, even today we learn from anatomy books and charts that were largely purged of connective tissue, and in which muscles with their well-defined contours appear more or less carved out. This results in easy-to-grasp maps of the body with boundaries that are as similarly arbitrary as those between countries and continents.

But the rivers of this world don't care. They flow beyond the borders made by men and travel long distances. And that is how it is inside the living body as well: Connective tissue is a hydrous, three-dimensional network that permeates the body in every direction, from top to bottom, from front to back, and from the outside to the inside.

This body-wide fiber network also isn't concerned with artificial anatomical boundaries. Only we humans seem to grasp this complex interconnectedness bit by bit. To quote the internationally renowned fascia researcher and anatomy professor Andry Vleemig, who recently proclaimed at one of his top-notch seminars: "Today we announce the new discovery that everything is connected by connective tissue. As if it had ever been separated."

From solid state to dynamic flow

As soon as the fascia loses its original wetness, the translucent membranes and shiny sheaths fundamentally change after just a few minutes. They lose their slipperiness, become brittle, and their formerly translucent color changes to an opaque white. A good example is the reticaculum, a fascial structure surrounding the ankle, that can only be viewed through a magnifier as it appears translucent. Exposure to air causes this collagen structure to harden and turn white, after which it resembles a tight plaster bandage like those in anatomical illustrations. This illustration has little in common with real life.

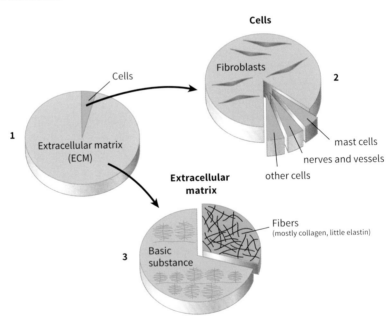

Fascia components: 1. Extracellular matrix (ECM) and connective-tissue cells. 2. The connective-tissue cells, particularly the fibroblasts, are the network's builders. Mast cells are responsible for immune defense. 3. The extracellular matrix consists of the basic substance and fibers. But most of the fascia is taken up by water.

This example suggests that we should change our conventional model of a solid body and instead recognize the significance of fluid processes. As soon as we take into account the connective tissue's fluid dynamics, chiropractors touch their clients differently, and exercise instructors apply different stimuli during training that stimulate the inner flow.

"The anatomical preparations in a medical classroom have as little in common with the juicy fascia of a living human as a dried raisin does with a fresh grape," says Robert Schleip, PhD.

New Information on a Well-Known Topic: Water

Have you ever asked yourself why Jell-O, which consists of 98% water, can be cut into solid cubes without flowing off the plate? Or why you can carefully place a 1-cent coin in a full glass of water and the surface tension is so stable that the coin won't sink?

A leading water researcher, Dr. Gerald Pollack (University of Washington), asked himself these same questions and his research findings are widely accepted by academic science. Previously calling oneself a water researcher was seen as almost dubious, and science relegated the impressive findings by some in alternative circles of well-respected water experts to the realm of intuition or wild speculation.

The fourth phase of water

In school we learned that water exists in three aggregate states: liquid, solid, and gas. Scientists who try to get on to this transient element and its peculiarities also knew that water molecules are also extremely eager to bond. But they can maintain their bonds for only a fraction of a second (approximately 10 nanoseconds). Gerald Pollack calls this form of water bulk water or unbound water.

Pollack proved that water molecules behave differently on negatively and positively charged surfaces: They enter into stable bonds and arrange themselves in a pattern over thousands of molecule layers. Therefore this form, or fourth phase, of water is referred to as structured water.

Exciting is that structured water is arranged just like a crystal, albeit a liquid crystal. Even more exciting is how this relates to connective tissue: Here approximately half of the water molecules are structured, creating liquid crystal. Healthy connective

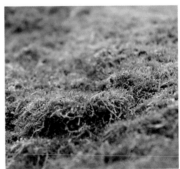

A healthy fascia is like fresh moss that is saturated with water, much like a sponge.

tissue is like luscious moss with countless dewdrops in its leaves. The water in dewdrops is structured water.

You can hold a piece of moss in your hand and it is wet and juicy. Only when you squeeze the moss does the water come out and you hold primarily fibers in your hand.

Fascial stasis: a sign of overload

Abnormal changes in the connective tissue are often characterized by unstructured water primarily in the tissue. Imagine the formerly luscious moss with individual or even extensive areas where water sits in a stagnant puddle. As you know: Dammed waters are not conducive to thriving.

Disturbances in the fluid dynamics within the human connective tissue can also cause swelling and edema. When edema form, it is a sign of overload. The described stagnation as well as the basic substance becoming more dense create a thickening and adhesiveness in the tissues, another sign of overloading.

Schleip, PhD, explains: "Imagine the notorious couch potato who goes for a run in his unfit state. Or someone whose knee has been in a cast for some time, and who decides on day one to walk down a long flight of stairs without the cast. And when his knee subsequently swells he may see this as confirmation that climbing stairs is harmful and should be avoided. But it would be smart if he were able to connect his knee's decreased load-bearing capacity with his previous lack of exercise and begin to reintroduce his knee to such load-bearing activities via healthy strengthening exercises."

When attempting to transform a previously brittle connective tissue into healthy, juicy tissue it is important to increase exercise intensity cautiously, consistently, and over an extended period of time. When remodeling fascia, the attitude "the harder the better" is outdated. Therefore, we recommend starting with caution and only low loading intensities that you then increase slowly over the upcoming weeks and months.

How easily we misjudge what an optimal load requirement should be. We can see this, among other things, in studies done on running in five finger shoes, a form of training in which each toe is individually encased in a very pared-down version of a shoe with a very thin sole. Runners who ignored the manufacturer's recommendation to wear the shoes for only 10 minutes after a run and continued to exercise in them showed more incidents of bone marrow edema than runners who wore conventional running shoes. This is interpreted as an overload symptom.

Conclusion: Definitely load fascial tissues, but do it the right way. Building healthy fiber networks requires constant attention and the attitude of a bamboo gardener: regular and patient care. More information on remodeling, meaning building permanently youthful elastic connective tissue, can be found in chapter 5.

Fibers, Fluid, and Cells

The components of fascia are cells and extracellular matrix (ECM). Extracellular matrix consists of fibers (primarily collagen) and a lesser amount of elastin fibers, as well as the so-called basic substance. A fascia consists mostly of water (68%), which forms a sticky blend of sugar-protein compounds and hyaluronic acid. This fluid, whose consistency and stickiness is similar to that of egg white, connects the body's structures, literally the connective tissue.

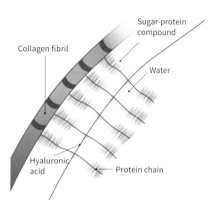

The extracellular matrix consists of collagen fibers, water-attracting sugar-protein compounds, and hyaluronic acid. The collagen fibril practically swims in an inner ocean whose sticky consistency is like that of egg albumen.

Water-attracting substances

Hyaluronan, the more accurate term for hyaluronic acid, is extremely hydrophilic, meaning it loves water. It absorbs 1000 times its own weight in water. If you add a tablespoon of hyaluronic acid to bathtub full of water, the water will gelatinize.

Attached to the collagen fiber is a hyaluronic acid chain where sugar-protein compounds that are also hydrophilic attach themselves. These structures look like small bottlebrushes whose bristles fan out and bind themselves to water in even the tiniest spaces.

Here again we can refer to the analogy to healthy moss which, when it is green and juicy, is saturated with water. But when metabolic waste, cellular waste, and free radicals accumulate in the basic substance the water bell collapses, resulting in puddles, stagnant areas in the tissue. Two things will help here: lots of exercise and a foam roller.

Hyaluronan, the magical substance?

One might think that lots of hyaluronan would be really good for the connective tissue. At least the cosmetics industry credits it with almost magical rejuvenating effects, and in sports medicine hyaluronic acid is also frequently used as a therapeutic tool for collagen injuries.

But people should remain skeptical because the question of whether or not the body can properly handle externally administered hyaluronic acid is currently being answered via a kind of field test on the paying consumer.

Italian anatomy professor Carla Stecco warns of administering non-endogenous hyaluronic acid. Her rationale: The externally administered substance may foster long molecular chains that cause thickening of the fluid film within the fibers. In a healthy state under the influence of hyaluronan, water acts as a lubricant for the fascia, allowing gliding and sliding. If this process is reversed, hyaluronan acts like a superglue, firmly sticking tissues together. Professor Stecco calls this process densification. In layman's terms, the hyaluronan acts like an adhesive.

Aging means dehydrating

On some level we are all fish, particularly at the beginning of our earthly existence, because newborns consist of more than 80% water and adults of at least 68%. In old age, the water content steadily decreases. An 80-year-old has only 50%. This means we increasingly dehydrate in the course of a long life. According to fascia researcher Schleip, PhD, this dehydration has several disadvantages for the connective tissue: "Aging is accompanied by two changes in the connective tissue. One, the water content significantly decreases, which results in more rigid tissue, making us less flexible. This causes a decrease in elasticity and makes the connective tissue more brittle. The result: Fibers tear more easily at the same tensile load intensity."

Contrary to past assumptions, drinking lots of fluids does little to, for instance, hydrate the Achilles tendon and other fascia. The effective strategy is mechanical stimulation like stretching and squeezing the sponge-like tissue with a foam roller.

Bouncing and skipping movements increase circulation and are particularly beneficial to the lymphatic flow, which in turn has a positive effect on the fluid dynamics. Stretching, as well as slow movements on the foam roller, squeezes the stagnant water out of the tissue. In return fresh water provided by the blood plasma flows back in.

Aging means crystallization

The second effect that significantly increases with age is the gradual formation of caramel-like crystals in the connective tissue's basic substance. This process can be compared to honey in a jar that has not been moved for a long period of time and crystallizes out at the edges.

In humans this caramelizing is also a natural and, to some extent, unstoppable progress. Experts refer to advanced glycation end products. As with honey it is possible to partly counteract this crystallization and the associated brittleness by regularly stirring the basic substance.

We can learn two things from honey: First, timing is important, because once the crystallization is too advanced even thorough stirring will result in only partial liquefaction. It is also important to reach hidden areas, meaning mechanical stimulation of even the most remote corners of our connective tissue. One of the ways we achieve this in fascia training is with lots of angle and directional changes in stretching positions or foam rolling.

In addition, lifestyle choices play an important part in connective tissue. Poor nutrition and the presence of stress hormones rocket the inflammation mediators and free radicals make mischief. This causes the basic substance to crystallize more quickly. "But even the highest-quality beekeeper's honey has to be stirred and liquefied because here, too, the process of crystallization is unstoppable. People with an optimal lifestyle (good stress management, clean air, a healthy diet) can get by with may be 15 to 30% less fascia training. But there is definitely no substitute," explains Robert Schleip, PhD.

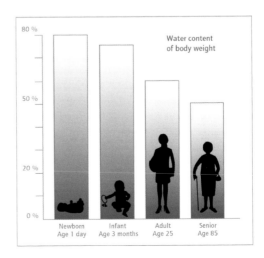

Newborns are more than 75% water. As we age the body's water content decreases (i.e., we dehydrate).

Self-Treatment: Foam Roller

Self-treatment with the foam roller has become quite popular and is in no way limited to the exclusive care of pro soccer players by innovative physical therapists. Nowadays lots of people roll in their living rooms. This is definitely a preferable trend, but using the foam roller takes some practice. In fascia training we use the foam roller in two different ways, each with a different effect. Following are the secrets to foam rolling.

Rolling for rehydration

To stimulate the fluid dynamics of the basic substance and to rehydrate tissue, it is recommended to slowly roll in different directions. You should plow through the tissue in a continuous motion with noticeable pressure all the way to "pleasurable" pain. Avoid quick back-and-forth movement in one spot or abrupt stop-and-go interruptions. The fluids should be moved thoroughly and the fascia sponges squeezed out. A frequently asked question in my classes is whether it is important to move in the direction of lymphatic flow. The answer is: You can do so if you want to specifically stimulate lymphatic drainage, but it is not absolutely necessary for rehydrating the tissue because 90% of the used water is released into the venous system and only 10% into the lymph. Since we are dealing with a wide network, fascia trainers recommend always rolling in different directions. This allows you to reach even the smallest of the tissue's branches and grooves. The foam roller's hardness is also not critical to the outcome, but the continuity of the rolling motion is important, and that can be achieved just as well with a softer roller. The good news: Filtered water streams from the blood plasma and refills the moss-like tissue with the positive effect of making the tissue fresher and juicier. An example of rehydration can be found in chapter 5.

Rolling for toning

We will now add another aspect to rolling training: fast and robust rolling. The purpose of this rolling treatment is not hydration but rather strengthening and toning the tissue. Fast and vigorous rubbing quickly increase the tissue's tonicity, which is important for performing dynamic or bouncing movements or for running. To do so, elastic fibers should have a high degree of tonicity, and this is achieved via brief, robust rolling at the start of training. Both rolling methods are used specifically as an anti-cellulite treatment. Slow rolling puts emphasis on squeezing mini edema and stagnant areas, stimulating fluid dynamics. Robust and fast rolling triggers mini tornadoes and turbulence within the basic which provoke the myofibroblasts to produce more collagen, reshaping the thigh. It is therefore acceptable to roll vigorously until there is pain.

Fibroblasts: sensitive little guys

One thing has puzzled researchers for a long time: How does a fibroblast, which speaks a biochemical language, recognize the purely mechanical stimulation that takes place, for instance in sports, or during a massage or treatment with a foam roller? Previously, specific receptor sites had been identified on the fibroblasts' cellular membranes with which the fibroblasts recognize mechanical forces and translate them into biochemical signals. However, their reaction is generally very sluggish. An exciting new discovery was the finding that to do so fibroblasts use cilia, tiny hair-like projections on their exterior as highly sensitive antennae.

These flexible feelers allow them to measure the speed of the surrounding fluid. To put it simply, they recognize if the fluid is moving very quickly or very slowly. During stormy seas, the fibroblasts strengthen and stabilize the networks. When the fluids are moving quickly, the fibroblasts strengthen the network by laying down more, stronger collagen fibers. Slower moving fluids soften the tissues and break down excess collagen. Fibroblasts are amazingly sensitive little guys.

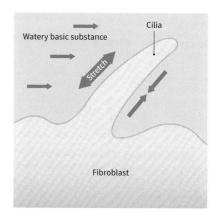

The cilia (tiny hair-like projections) allow the connective tissue cell to feel into the fluid dynamics of the surrounding basic substance. Depending on the flow rate, it synthesizes or breaks down collagen.

Self-Treatment: Cupping Therapy

Cupping therapy to improve connective tissue has been a common practice for decades. This method can appear somewhat outdated and doesn't look particularly sexy. Nevertheless, the suction cup is able to do something the roller cannot: The suction creates a vacuum resulting in traction, specifically between the subcutaneous tissue and the fascia profunda, the body's catsuit. When the cup is pulled across the skin adhesions and adherences are released.

We can also assume that suction cup therapy boosts the local circulation and metabolism with a positive effect on the connective tissue. A study also verified that the fast and vigorous application of suction cup therapy promotes collagen synthesis and remodeling. For this reason we also use this tried-and-proven tool for toning and especially for cellulite treatments.

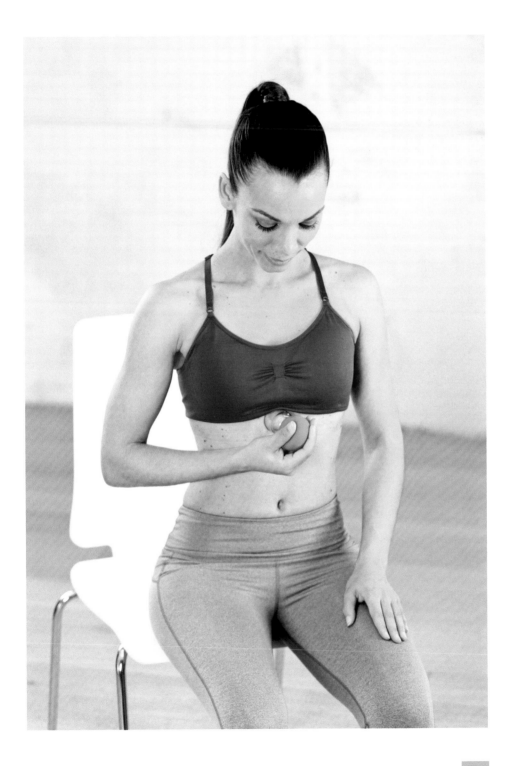

4 Show Me Your Connective Tissue and I'll Tell You Your Age

Some people don't show their age. Fortunately that has nothing to do with Botox or cosmetic surgery, but with the fact that these people have exercised all of their lives.

We women can be self-conscious about our face and skin, and our first wrinkles cause us to ponder our age. But studies show that it is the overall impression that determines whether we find someone attractive and youthful. What matters is an upright posture, supple movements, and a light-footed gait. Approving comments like "That woman looks amazing for her age" or "That man is a regular spring chicken" indicate that there are factors other than our genes that impact our mobility and vitality.

On that point, there is good news from the connective tissue department. Danish researchers state that with adequate exercise connective tissue in older adults can be rejuvenated by up to 20 years. That means a 60-year-old woman cannot regain the body of a 20-year-old, but can be as elastic and springy as a 40-year-old. That is motivating and suggests that the secret of youth can be achieved through fascia training.

Nature or nurture?

The debate over whether our health is predetermined by our genes or whether the influences of environment, upbringing, and attitude play a greater role is not new. But today there is a general consensus that we are much more malleable, meaning pliable, as adults than was previously thought. The things that shape us in the course of our lives—

our experiences, our relationships, the way we handle life's small and big challenges— shape our body, spirit, and psyche in positive and negative ways.

The connective tissue also provides a rich source of plasticity. There is the older woman who spent years training for marathons, practiced gymnastics or yoga, or did yard work in all kinds of weather. Or the older man who spent every free moment hiking in the mountains, enjoyed sitting by a campfire at night, and forwent the comforts of a soft hotel bed to sleep in a tent instead. Such activities promote versatility, strength, and mobility, and work on coordination, muscles, and fascia, while couch potatoes do not sufficiently utilize their genetic disposition for walking and running, squatting and climbing, but rather let it atrophy. Their true age isn't just in their bones but also in their connective tissue. The expression "nature or nurture" really gets to the heart of the interplay between inherent abilities on the one hand, and life and learning history on the other hand. Because what we do with our abilities really comes down us.

In this context connective tissue plasticity refers to training, nutrition, and lifestyle. We already explained that serious illnesses, injuries, accidents, and surgeries affect connective tissue function. But just like our emotional attitude, traumatic events and sustained stress also impact the flexibility and resilience of our fascia.

"A person's level of flexibility and vitality is not only determined by his genes but also by exercise and upbringing," says Robert Schleip, PhD. "We should therefore be creative and seize as many everyday opportunities to feed our natural urge to move and our biological mandate for physical challenges (i.e., to return to a Homo sapiens' species-appropriate attitude)."

Use It or Lose It

Four questions to Robert Schleip, PhD

1. Why is it so important for us to mechanically load our bodies?

    Robert Schleip, PhD: "The catchphrase 'Use it or lose it' is a perfect expression. This quote harkens back to the 19th century Wolff's law about bone health. Actual studies done with astronauts show that bones, which are also connective tissue, drastically atrophy when astronauts are unable to move properly during their space travels due to the lack of gravitational pull. But with adequate loading the bone will synthesize and strengthen."

2. How does connective tissue react when it is insufficiently loaded?

    Robert Schleip, PhD: "Here the so-called Davis law applies. The American orthopedist Henry Gassett Davis transferred Wolff's law on bones to the fibrous connective tissue and found that the same principle applies. The fibrous connective tissue that includes the tendons also becomes brittle and fragile when it is not loaded sufficiently.

    But when we challenge the fascia, it becomes stronger. However, you should not over-exercise because that will weaken the fascia. This principle is called mechano-adaption, or simply "Use it or lose it."

3. What would you recommend to people of the Viking type?

    Robert Schleip, PhD: "These people are generally quite stiff and sturdy, but have limited flexibility and stretching ability. For Viking types, it is of particular interest that regular stretching exercises and proper fascia training can make them more flexible; melting stretches are particularly beneficial. In addition, Viking types can modify their strength training to specifically exhaust the muscles in the end range position. The body then gets the message to reorganize so that its new middle, or rather its new working range, is in this stretched-out load area. In other words, the muscle tissue and fascia begin to adapt to a new length in that area."

4. What type of training would you recommend for the temple dancer types?

    Robert Schleip, PhD: "Here we recommend working the muscle and its fascial sheath specifically in the area where the loaded muscle fibers are shortened the most. The body then gets the message to adapt the length of the loaded myofascial tissue over weeks and months so that the muscle's new middle shifts towards the short area. This allows the tissue to firm up and become more toned."

Coach Potatoes

"Sitting for four hours is just as bad as smoking one pack of cigarettes a day." This assertion by the renowned American oncologist David Agus packs a punch because we have long known about the harmful effects of nicotine. But why does Agus compare smoking to sitting for hours on end? Are couch potatoes just as bad off as smokers? As you read this, you may be sitting in an armchair, at your kitchen table, or on a park bench. Maybe you take a small break to stretch for a few minutes while you read. And if you really think about it, you may have been sitting since you got up in the morning and after closing this book you could take a bike ride or go for a brisk walk or run.

The expression "going into retirement" is quite revealing, because it suggests that we want to downshift, take it easy, and just laze around.

But Homo sapiens are built to move. Early man (Homo erectus) walked 6+ miles every day. Until about 50 years ago, it was common to walk as much as 12 miles a day. Current research sadly shows that modern man walks only about 300 steps a day. We have to therefore ask ourselves: Did evolution go through all this trouble of putting humans at the top of creation only so they can shuffle 300 steps to buy the next pack of cigarettes? In short, sitting for hours on end is bad for us.

Sitting is rigid posture and mostly motionless. Overdoing it and sitting without taking breaks is bad for the tissue and causes inflammation parameters to go up. Our connective tissue gets brittle and causes us to age more rapidly. "The debate over couch potatoes is boiling up everywhere and has not yet reached its climax because just like the debate over smoking, it is not a fad," explains fascia researcher Robert Schleip, PhD. "Scientific data even shows that the consequences are much worse than expected."

The sad thing about sitting for hours on end is that the tissue damage is only partially repairable. "Part of the tissue damage can be corrected via targeted fascia training. A half hour of movement after sitting for four hours helps the tissue, but it is not enough or is too late to fully compensate for the health-related metabolic disadvantages caused by prolonged inertia. This new finding surprised and shocked me as well," says Robert Schleip, PhD. The debate over nicotine has changed society more than some researchers anticipated. Robert Schleip, PhD: "In a nutshell, sitting is the new smoking. Hopefully when enough people and institutions recognize this, it could possibly change our society's culture as fundamentally as has already happened in recent years with the smoking culture at the work place and in restaurants."

If you have to sit a lot, get up occasionally!

When you sit at a desk from morning to evening, it makes sense to think about what opportunities you may have to occasionally stand up and move around:

- Don't call your colleague in the adjacent office, but walk over to her.

- Make a date with a colleague for a tea or coffee break at a specific time.

- Take a walk around the block during your lunch break.

- Use a lectern for making phone calls or taking notes.

- Work at a hydraulically adjustable desk that has a timer attached to it.

- Skip the elevator and walk, or better yet skip, up and down the steps.

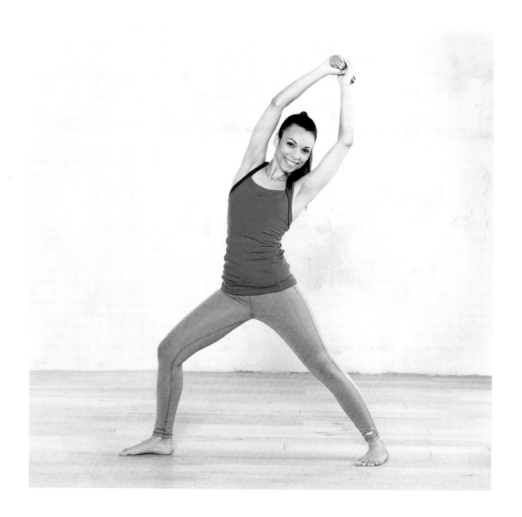

Overloaded or Underloaded?

Question to Robert Schleip, PhD

Why are so many people physically underloaded?

Robert Schleip, PhD: "Many people believe the human body is like a car that suffers pain when the tires are abraded by the road asphalt. But the body is a biological organism that continuously adapts to the interaction with its environment. When it is insufficiently challenged, its resilience rapidly declines. If we then take the car for a spin, it is overburdened because the tissue has become thin. Since most people don't have a variety of physical activity in their daily lives, this will not improve in the long term since we avoid any additional physical effort. Ideally people should build a variety of physical activities into their daily lives so the tissue doesn't atrophy."

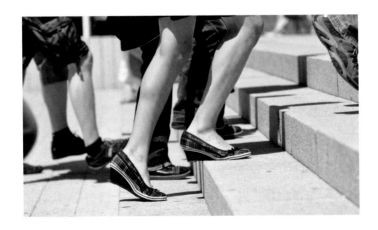

Human Species-Appropriate Movement

When a dolphin is in his element, he will swim up to 124 miles a day through the ocean. If he were kept in a bathtub, someone would immediately call the humane society to release him from his prison even if the bathtub was made of gold, the dolphin was fed the best food, and had relaxing music playing in the background. Because none of that helps! When the species-appropriate movement is missing, the liver, brain, and lymph system can no longer fully function.

There are other examples from the animal kingdom. When whales that were kept for years in large pools by us humans were released into the ocean, they often perished miserably. The reason: If the transition from lack of movement to surviving freely in the ocean is too rapid, it can also be deadly.

Often we are also like caged tigers because we no longer get a species-appropriate amount of exercise. But as tempting as it may be to quickly leave our civilized cage, we too must slowly adapt to the challenges of a natural, physically active lifestyle.

Hunter-gatherers

To find out which conditions must be met for a human's species-appropriate lifestyle, researchers looked into the questions: How did prehistoric man spend his days? How did Stone Age people move? And what do we know about the tribal cultures of hunter-gatherers still living today in Mexico and Africa? One answer is simple: All of them were much more active than we are today.

Running, throwing, climbing, and squatting—anyone who does these things for hours every day builds his endurance, strength, and flexibility. In spite of their physically active lives, our ancestors' average calorie consumption was not much higher than ours is today. That means most modern humans eat too much and move too little.

Evolutionary medicine is a special field in which renowned physicians and scientists work to learn about our contemporary health problems. The timeline clearly shows that four billion years of natural history are followed by only five million years since the dawn of mankind. But since the Stone Age, hunter-gatherers had to rapidly adapt to constantly evolving environmental conditions without their bodies being able to keep up in all its functions.

But how can we return to moving in a species-appropriate way? Fascia researchers like Robert Schleip, PhD, and his colleague Edo Hemar recommend walking, climbing, pushing, and pulling, as well as lifting, carrying, squatting, and throwing as primary species-appropriate human moves. Innovative fitness instructors create various functional exercises such as Primary Movement, Paleo Fitness, Evo Fitness, or MovNat.

Walking and running

Chimpanzees can take only a few steps in an upright position, and they are not really able to walk fast but that would not be an advantage in the dense jungle. But walking on two legs makes a lot of sense when hunting on the steppe. No wonder our ancestors developed into bipeds and long-distance runners.

Walking is considered the supreme discipline of human locomotion because we are perfectly suited for it. Even back in the Stone Age, the toes were shortened so our ancestors were better able to roll the foot heel to toe. At the lower calf the springy elastic fascia connects to the Achilles tendon, a human's thickest and strongest tendon. The connective tissue band at the bottom of the foot, the plantar fascia, supports us from below during our springy walk. Mother Nature made sure that we are hard to beat as endurance runners. We are able to run down almost any animal, one of the hunting methods of our ancestors.

Our long Achilles tendons make it possible for us to run as light-footed as a gazelle, jump like a kangaroo, and leap like a cat. To do so, the tendons and fascia of the legs are prestretched like elastic rubber bands. When the tendons and fascia are let loose, the stored energy is released, enabling the leaping motion.

Find out in the practical part of the book beginning in chapter 5, how you can train for this elastic, or catapult effect.

The rediscovered barefoot or minimalist-shoe culture

"Nature did not forget the invention of shoes but rather gave us feet." This quote is from Harvard University's distinguished anthropologist Daniel Lieberman, who is also known as the barefoot professor. In his lab he researches, among other things, the effects of modern cushioned running shoes compared to running barefoot. Lieberman, who has himself become a firm believer in running barefoot, found that runners who wear high-tech running shoes tend to land on the heel and then roll onto the ball of the foot. For many years, fitness instructors and running coaches taught this heel striking method as the optimal running technique.

When Lieberman and his team put experienced barefoot runners on the treadmill, they were surprised to find that they naturally landed on the front of the foot, called forefoot striking. The barefoot runner's initial contact with the ground is made with the fourth to fifth metatarsal bone, then rolls onto the big toe, and finally onto the heel.

Lieberman and his colleague, renowned sports medicine specialist Dr. Irene Davis, proved that in forefoot runners the ground reaction force has less impact on knee and hip joints. Both therefore suspect that for many runners gradually switching to a barefoot-like running style could be healthier for their knee and hip joints.

Back to nature?

All of the statements about species-appropriate movement might tempt one to start living based on the motto "Back to nature." Throw out your chairs, kick your running shoes to the curb, and entrust yourself completely to your evolutionary heritage. But be forewarned: The feet of barefoot walkers who walk long distances have practiced this from childhood and possess extraordinary elasticity and strength.

If your feet grew up in a shoe prison, it is best to start with a few barefoot steps at the end of a regular run. If that goes well, you can slowly increase the amount weekly.

It is fine to go back to nature, but we must do so with common sense and reason, and most of all enduring patience, otherwise overload damage and injuries are inevitable. Plan for at least one year to transform your degenerate civilization foot into a strong and elastic paw like that of a barefoot walker. Increase your hip mobility over the course of weeks and months by frequently and regularly sitting and squatting on the floor, initially for a short time, and gradually for longer. You can find exercises to strengthen your feet beginning in chapter 5 of this book.

Climbing and moving hand-over-hand

Chimpanzees living in a non-species-appropriate environment at a zoo surprisingly suffer from similar forms of arthrosis as humans. Anthropologist Dr. Robert McNeill Alexander followed large apes in the wild, filmed their joint movements, and compared his findings to human movement behavior.

During analysis he realized that the joints we use in a very limited way as compared to our fellow species are very often affected by arthrosis as well as rheumatic degeneration, while the joints we use in an ape-like manner stay as healthy as those in apes that live in a species-appropriate environment.

Based on this information, the researcher developed the unused arc theory. The supposition: Limited loading promotes degenerative processes such as rheumatism and arthritis because arthrosis. The interesting find was that degeneration doesn't start in the loaded areas but rather in the unused edges of the joint's pathway because of poor metabolic activity.

Robert Schleip, PhD, explains this principal via an example: "A door can be opened 180 degrees. But when we use only 90 degrees or less to walk through it may happen that the hinges will only move freely within that limited range. Over the course of months, deposits and dirt collect in the unused peripheral areas so that at some point the door will no longer open all the way. In our daily lives we mostly use our shoulder mobility to pull our hanging arms into a horizontal position. That's maximally 90 degrees. We only use the remaining 270 degrees when we pull on a sweater. Thus the shoulder joint is only rarely exposed to tensile and compressive loading in this unused area."

For this reason, the participants of our fascial fitness classes play on playgrounds. They practice moving hand-over-hand, hanging upside-down, and other monkey-like movements on the monkey bars. Here our shoulder joints are finally in full use again and the world is upside-down. During this activity in the "monkey gym," the fascial tissues around the muscles are optimally toned in the short-range position through optimal loading and optimal toning.

As soon as the participants have crossed the "adults don't do that" threshold they have loads of fun. Their initial skepticism changes to laughing faces and sparkling eyes.

Squatting and sitting

Are you familiar with the sculpture of eight squatting Chinese figures in Bamberg, Germany? The sculpture of male figures painted red caused quite a stir in 2014, when it was installed. Barefoot and with their legs apart they squat in a circle, arms between knees and hands on the grass.

We possess a distinct seating furniture culture; we rarely get down on the floor but rather lounge or sprawl many hours each day on chairs, armchairs, or sofas. For our bodies, the invention of the chair is non-physiological and it is no wonder that the back aches, the hip joints freeze up, and the muscles at the back of the legs shorten. In Asian countries, it is still completely natural to squat on the floor. There people sit for hours at the market, the bus stop, and the hole-in-the-ground latrine.

For children it is usually still easy to completely fold the ankles, knee, and hip joints, but the older we get the more difficult it is to get into that bunny posture.

Muslims probably still have less trouble getting into a squat since they must kneel and bend over several times a day for prayers. "For many people sitting on the floor and squatting is not easy," cautions Robert Schleip, PhD. "Their calf muscles have shortened so severely over the years that they cannot get low enough. Many can only do so while wearing high heels."

Everyday exercises: sitting and squatting variations

Frequently change your sitting position during your daily routine, for instance while eating, reading, or during your lunch break:

- Cross-legged seat: Don't sit in a chair but rather on the floor on a tatami mat or a cushion.

- Heel sit: Kneel on the floor and sit back on your heels, while keeping your trunk upright.

- Child's pose: In a heel sit, bend forward and rest your head in front of your knees. In yoga this child's pose is often used as a relaxing closing pose.

The deep squat position is a part of our fascia training. You can view this basic position on page 100. It will help you to sit in a joint-friendly manner on the floor at home or in the grass at the park. Doing this once a day is a good start. By doing our dynamic exercises like the frog jump you will find that it gradually gets easier over the weeks and months.

Throwing and hurling

A little evolutionary guessing game: Do you know what differentiates the Australopithecus who lived four to two million years ago in Africa from his successor, Homo erectus?

One of the criteria identified by paleoanthropologists from Professor Daniel Lieberman's research group was the impressive physical ability that Homo erectus developed for throwing. His skeleton changed so much that the upright human was able to walk on two legs and could also rotate his shoulder extremely fast. "Next to a wider range of motion, the fascial components in the respective parts of the body needed for throwing apparently also contributed to this," says Robert Schleip, PhD. "A considerable amount of the kinetic energy is provided by dynamic elastic capacity, the catapult effect of fascia." So we can add throwing as an originally species-appropriate movement to the impressive storage capacity of the Achilles tendon that made us into bipedal animals. To build strong and flexible shoulders, it therefore makes sense to integrate throwing into our weekly schedules. Dog owners who throw sticks might have an advantage here.

There are a few other everyday options:

- Toss a ball or Frisbee back and forth with a partner in a variety of ways.

- You can do partner juggling exercises by throwing the balls, pins, and rings over your head.

- Try javelin or discus throwing.

- Try our throwing exercises in the practical part of the book.

Connective Tissue Nourishment

It is better to exercise and not have an optimal diet than to eat strictly organic food but lie on the couch all day. "The fascia is more sensitive to over- and underloading during mechanical stimulation than to nutrition," explains Robert Schleip, PhD. While exercising regularly and correctly is essential for a healthy fascia, you can additionally nourish your connective tissue with the right nutrition.

But which diet is particularly beneficial to the fascia? Unfortunately there is no scientifically founded answer at this time, and scientific studies on the subject are still scarce. Nutritional research continues to gain new insights that disprove previously accepted assertions, and besides, when it comes to a healthy diet many contradictory opinions already circulate.

All that doesn't make it easy to make comprehensive recommendations for a fascia-friendly diet, but we do hope that the diligently working fascia researchers will be able to contribute solid results on this exciting topic in the foreseeable future.

Right now we can get behind one guideline: A diet that keeps down inflammation in the body is a fascia-friendly diet. "To date there are no studies that prove that an anti-inflammatory diet definitely improves connective tissue health," explains Robert Schleip, PhD. "However, we can refer to the nutritional studies on rheumatoid diseases in which inflammation of the muscles and fascia including tendons and joints can occur. They give us possible clues to the right fascial nutrition in healthy people."

By the way, you will not yet get any results from an Internet search under the keyword "fascial nutrition" because to date only a few fascia and nutrition researchers have spoken about it publicly. Nevertheless, in this book we tackle the subject and hope to initiate more in-depth and conclusive cooperation across disciplines.

What is inflammation?

As unpleasant as it can be, inflammation is a way for our body to defend itself against pathogens by fighting them. During the complicated healing process, cell residue accumulates that must be broken down so the affected areas can recover and regenerate.

The following five symptoms are typical for inflammation: redness, heat, swelling, pain, and restricted movement.

1. Increased perfusion results in redness in affected areas.

2. The affected area is warm; fever can also be a symptom of internal inflammation.

3. Swelling occurs because fluid from blood accumulates.

4. When edema push on nerves, we feel pain.

5. When something hurts we often tend to put as little weight as possible on it and try not to move it.

Please note: In order to explain the possible effects of nutrition on inflammation as simply as possible, we will refer to terminology by nutrition expert Dr. Michaela Döll and compare inflammation to a fire:

- It all begins with the fire starter.

- The inflamed areas are the fire sources and fireplaces.

- The *good* anti-inflammatory foods are fire extinguishers.

- The *bad* foods are fire accelerants that contribute to worsening inflammation.

To avoid burdening the tissue and metabolism with inflammation, nutritionists recommend consuming fire extinguishers and forgoing fire accelerants.

Fire starters: belly fat is bad

We often hear that being overweight is bad. But what does that mean with regard to the connective tissue? The BMI (body mass index) is not well-suited for answering this question because it only focuses on height and weight. Much more important is the area of the body where fat accumulates. To be precise, we are talking about belly fat.

Doctors refer to fatty tissue on the belly, but especially in the belly, as visceral fat, meaning belonging to the intestines. Overweight people with a high BMI have a lot of visceral fat, but people with a medium BMI can also have visceral fat accumulating between the internal organs. The problem: Messengers that act as fire starters can become fire sources continuously forming in belly fat, resulting in potentially chronic inflammation of the tissue.

So what to do? Liposuction of excess belly fat would hardly work because surgeons are not able to reach the tissue surrounding the organs. You should exercise regularly and not take in more calories than you can burn.

The "drink a lot of fluids" myth

The myth that drinking a lot of fluids will thoroughly moisten the connective tissue has already been done away with in chapter 3. Tissue rehydration is largely achieved via mechanical stimulation such as foam rolling. Nutrition experts recommend that athletes drink as soon as they begin to feel thirsty, but not large quantities of water in a short period of time which can cause damage by washing out minerals. Drink sufficiently when you feel slightly thirsty. You can also intake fluids in the form of raw fruits and vegetables or soup.

Fire extinguishers: a list of good foods

At the top of the what-to-eat list is Jell-O. It consists primarily of gelatin, which is obtained mostly from pork rind and thus is cooked collagen.

American biologist Keith Baar speculates that the consumption of gelatin lessens the risk of injury in athletes. He was able to show in a cell culture that artificial ligaments became more tear-resistant when adding essential nutrients from gelatin. He therefore recommends eating a portion of Jell-O prior to exercising.

It is best to cook the Jell-O from an unsweetened gelatin and add some fruit juice or Stevia as a sweetener. Gummy bears will work, too, but a 7-ounce bag of gummy bears contains 3.2 ounces of sugar, the equivalent of 30 sugar cubes.

If you prefer it savory, you should try aspic, jus, cured meat in gelatin, and corned beef, because salt is less harmful to the fascia than sugar. Unfortunately, there is no alternative to gelatin for vegetarians and vegans because plants do not contain collagen. That is also why the respective nutritional supplements are made from animal products.

Fascia-friendly trace elements

Zinc ranks at the top of the list of fascia-friendly trace elements. It is present in the walls of the fascia, assists collagen production, and supports tissue repair. That is also the reason zinc ointment is used against and for treatment of sunburn.

It makes sense that we should also provide our bodies sufficient amounts of zinc internally. Top-ranked foods for zinc content are oysters and mussels, but beef and pork liver, crab, and cheese also contain lots of zinc. The body doesn't absorb this trace element as well from plant-based foods, but the requirements of vegans can be well met with lentils, soybeans, sunflower seeds, whole grains, and wheat bran.

Fascia-friendly enzymes

Bromelain is comprised of two enzymes that can be found in the trunk of the pineapple plant. This enzyme mix accelerates the healing process in cases of inflammation and reduces swelling more quickly. Bromelain can be extracted from the woody stalk of the pineapple.

Papain is present in papaya fruit, is anti-inflammatory, and is especially concentrated in the still-green, unripe fruit and its black seeds.

Chymotrypsin and trypsin are pancreatic juice enzymes and are mostly found in pork products. They also affect the fascia's disposition to inflammation and speed up tissue repair.

Plant- or animal-based fascia-friendly enzymes inhibit pro-inflammatory cytokines in the tissue. You can use enzymes as a course of treatment or as a preventative, but also for existing inflammation and to accelerate tissue repair. If you're not ready to fire up the juicer every day, you can also purchase prefabricated compounds. These consist of a mixture of the previously listed plant and animal enzymes. Of note is that, when necessary, a high-quality enzyme preparation can be combined with anti-inflammatory medications such as acetylsalicylic acid or diclofenac.

In the longer term, medications could potentially be replaced with a milder enzyme treatment, provided enzymes are taken properly; enzymes will take effect in the connective tissue when consumed ½ hour before or 2 hours after a meal. When taken with a meal, they merely break down the food in a highly efficient manner.

Vitamins

Vitamins A, E, and C, as well as beta-carotene as a precursor to vitamin A are antioxidants. We will detail them here with the addition of vitamin D.

Vitamin A can be found in liver, fish, milk, and cheese. You can meet your daily beta-carotene requirements primarily with carrots, but also with spinach, tomatoes, broccoli, and apricots. The body absorbs the provitamin A best when taken with a small amount of fat like, for instance, olive oil. Vitamin E, derived from plant oils, protects cell membranes and absorbs free radicals.

Vitamin C is important to connective tissue because it helps to hold the fibers together like an adhesive. Fennel, kale, broccoli, and red peppers are particularly high in vitamin C. Black currants, rosehips, and Acerola cherries are also considered vitamin C bombs.

Vitamin D reduces the amount of protein (cytokines) involved in inflammatory processes. This fat-soluble vitamin can be found primarily in cod-liver oil, herring, sardines, and salmon, but can also be found in smaller amounts in milk, eggs, and shitake mushrooms. However, sunlight is the most effective source of vitamin D. When we spend a lot of time outside (without sun protection), our body generally synthesizes sufficient amounts on its own. But here we must take into account the fact that sun exposure also increases the risk of skin cancer.

During the darker months it can be useful to take a vitamin D supplement. In this case – and when taking nutritional supplements in general – it is advisable to consult your physician. He can recommend suitable preparations and where necessary, monitor the intake. Doctors who practice alternative medicine often specialize in orthomolecular medicine, meaning the therapeutic use of dietary supplements.

Antioxidants

During inflammation there is an increase of free radicals in the body. Keeping these aggressive substances in check requires more free-radical interceptors. Antioxidants from fruits and vegetables play an important role here, particularly red goji berries from Asia. Anti-inflammatory carotenoids—the antioxidant plant compound anthocyanin in cherries, papaya, and blueberries—is also well-suited to neutralizing free radicals.

Onions and garlic contain sulfur compounds that support the immune system in its fight against pathogens. The antioxident quercetin also helps the body defend itself against inflammatory processes. Polyphenols are secondary plant compounds that act as antioxidants because they intercept free radicals in the body and are thereby able to protect the body from inflammation. Plants contain polyphenols in the form of pigments and flavoring substances as well as tanning agents.

The blue acai berries from the Brazilian jungle palm have a particularly high content of secondary plant compounds: 3.5 ounces contain approximately 135 milligrams of polyphenols.

Many plants contain precious polyphenols. Here are a variety of particularly potent substances for the connective tissue. Leading the way is the shrub yellow root, curcuma. Curcuma is an important ingredient in curry powders. Curcuma is particularly effective when it is ingested together with black pepper. This combination increases the anti-inflammatory effects sevenfold. Prepared blends in the form of capsules are available in stores and it is recommended to take 6 to 8 grams per day. It is best to gradually adjust to these quantities. To avoid stomach upset, capsules can be taken with yogurt.

Green tea and the epicatechin contained therein is another potent antioxident. If you don't want to drink gallons of green tea, you can also take green tea capsules or as matcha powder available in teashops. You can put a spoonful in a green morning smoothie, but remember that green tea has lots of caffeine and will wake you up, so don't take it late in the day if you want to be able to sleep at night.

Chili with the effective ingredient capsaicin is also a favorite fascial food. Special receptors in the connective tissue respond to the capsaicin. This substance is therefore also added to analgesic gels and crèmes, and helps with sports injuries like sprains, strains, or back pain. Capsaicin supplies the tissue with blood and warms the tissue locally, and in addition has a soothing effect on the irritated pain receptors. But be careful! Keep your hands away from your eyes after applying the crème, or they will burn terribly.

If you want to take capsaicin, you should increase the dose slowly, because capsaicin is extremely spicy.

Cacao and the flavanones contained therein are many people's favorite antioxidant in the form of dark chocolate. Please make sure the cacao content is at least 70% and the sugar content is as low as possible. It's worth a peek at the list of ingredients because sometimes the trusting consumer is led astray. Meanwhile there are many high-quality chocolate varieties available in the organic foods section at your grocery store or at the organic market.

Divo's favorite smoothie

Ingredients

- 1 avocado
- 1 pear
- ½ bunch of parsley
- 6-7 oz. of water

- 2 celery stalks
- 1 head of baby romaine lettuce
- ½ tsp. matcha powder
- 1 pinch of pepper

Preparation

Cut the avocado in half, remove the pit, and remove the flesh with a spoon. Wash the celery and cut it up. Wash the pear, quarter it, and remove the core. Wash the lettuce and parsley, remove excess water, and cut them up. Put all the ingredients in a blender, add matcha powder and water, and blend until smooth.

Add pepper to taste.

Omega-3 fatty acids

Fish oil contains lots of omega-3 fatty acids that have an anti-inflammatory effect. We recommend in particular fatty cold-water fish like herring, mackerel, salmon, and tuna, but rapeseed, flaxseed, and walnut oils also contain anti-inflammatory fatty acids.

Fire accelerators: a list of bad foods

Sweets are at the top of the pyramid of foods that cause inflammation. The sugar they contain is so harmful that we should eat as little of it as possible. Grain products that contain gluten, dairy and eggs can also have an inflammatory effect.

Oxidized fats also act as fire accelerants. Light and heat transform fats and oils so they can react more quickly with atmospheric oxygen. When they are stored in a light and warm place, the oxidation causes them to get rancid. Oxidized fats are also created during frying and grilling and, as fire accelerators, promote inflammation and tissue changes. Tip: Store fats and oils in a dark, cool place.

Sugar Causes Connective Tissue to Stiffen

A question to Robert Schleip, PhD

Most people consume too much sugar, and that doesn't just cause weight gain but also causes the skin and connective tissue to age more quickly. Why is sugar so bad for our bodies?

Robert Schleip, PhD: "The older we get, the more sugary we get. In the process, large crystal structures form in the connective tissue, causing it to get brittle. But we can slow down or speed up this crystallization process with the appropriate measures. An overly sweet diet promotes caramelization of the connective tissue. When you decrease your consumption of sugar and sugar-like carbohydrates and get a lot of exercise, you can slow down that process."

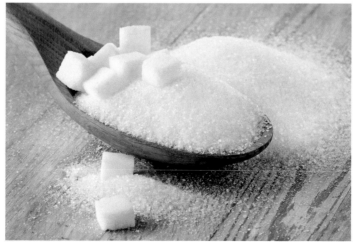

Too much of a good thing can also be bad. This is true for oils made from sunflower, corn, and safflower oils. These oils contain omega-6 fatty acids, which the body can use to create messengers that promote inflammation. When using a lot of oils it is best to fall back on rapeseed, walnut, and flaxseed oil.

Conclusion

You can take care of your fascia with fascia-friendly foods as well as specific nutritional supplements, and lower your inflammation markers. This is particularly advisable during times of high physical and mental stress because stress increases the body's disposition to inflammation and damages your connective tissue.

Nevertheless, nutrition is only a concomitant and supporting measure. The best therapy for healthy and toned connective tissue is exercise.

And that is what the practical part of the book is about. Let the fascia training begin!

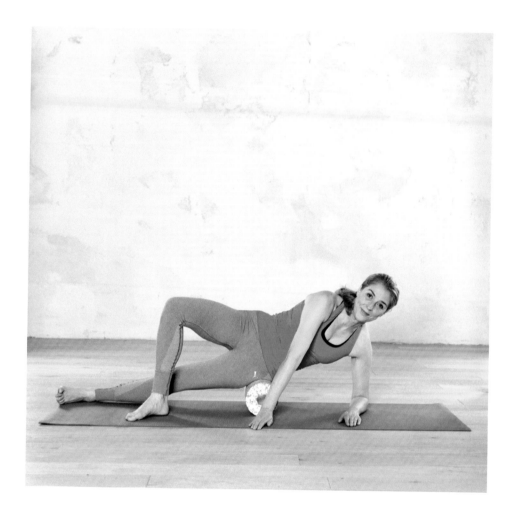

PRACTICE

Fascia Training

And now we will begin fascia training with lots of enthusiasm and vigor! You are now very familiar with the theoretical content, and you already know the most important fascia that we will strengthen and tighten with this exercise program.

If you took the self-test in chapter 2 and found out that individual fascia chains might require more flexibility, you can still complete the training. You will need to lengthen these fascia chains at the end of the training unit. You can find the respective practical explanation on pages 94-95.

First, we will introduce the basic elements of fascia training and then explain the specific method to tighten the connective tissue—our success formula. We will show you a number of exercises for each fascia chain to help build or regain strong elasticity for vital resilience, and last but not least, a toned body contour.

Have fun moving!

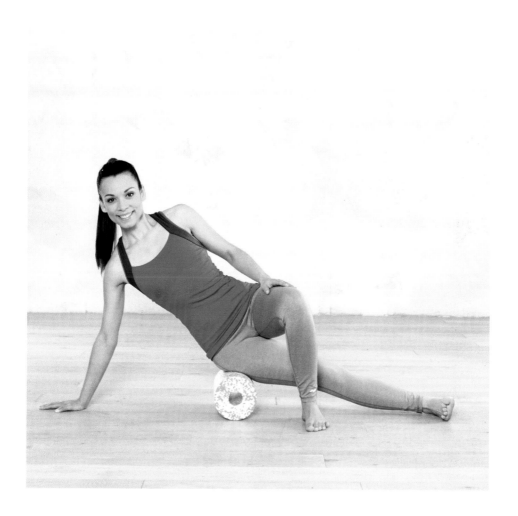

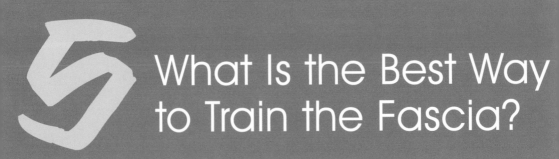

5 What Is the Best Way to Train the Fascia?

Exercise science has long underestimated the importance of the fascia, the muscular connective tissue, but current findings by international fascia researchers clearly show that connective tissue plays a major role in load transmission and builds an important foundation for flexibility, elasticity, and performance capacity. So we are not talking about an insignificant tissue, particularly since the body-wide collagen network is equipped with many stretch receptors and thus represents our most important sensory organ for body sense, proprioception. The fascia participates in every movement and contribute to back pain as well as physical well-being.

The basic fascial-fitness exercises can be integrated into preventative health programs, holistic approaches, and medical rehabilitation, as well as training for performance athletes. Likely in the future targeted strengthening of the fascia will play an important role in any serious training approach, meaning every training approach will include a fascia component.

In this section we will introduce one basic fascia exercise for each of the four categories of fasical training.

Targeted connective-tissue exercises have many benefits.

- The elastic collagen network serves as a natural prophylaxis for sports injuries. Most sports injuries are not muscular, but rather are the result of overloading the collagen tissue.

- The contribution of resilient connective tissue to a strong and healthy back has long been underestimated.

- "Feeling good in your skin" should really be "Feeing good in your fascia," because as a sensory organ, the collagen network greatly contributes to our well-being.

- As long as our muscular connective tissue is intact, our vitality is ensured as we get older. We remain flexible, our movements are smooth, and we literally move through life with a spring in our step.

- Movements that are controlled by the fascia, such as jumps and throws, are more efficient while at the same time give the impression of effortlessness and supple elegance.

- An important bonus: The fascia gives the body support and shape. When exercised properly, they provide healthy muscle tone and a beautifully defined body contour.

That last point is the aim of this book because shaping the body requires specific training principles. On page 95 we begin to lay out our success formula developed specifically to tighten connective tissue.

To do the training, you will need a variety of tools (like the ankle weights shown in the photo below); under "Tools and Tips" on page 176 you'll find resources and product information.

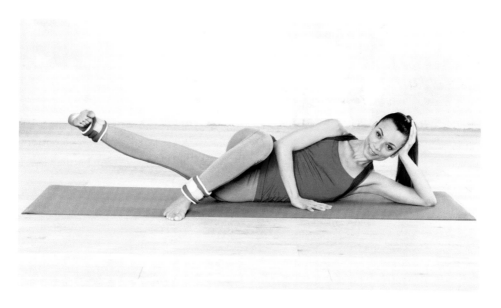

Tools for Fascia Training

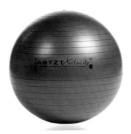

Large stability ball

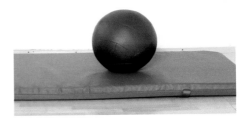

ATX CrossFit ball

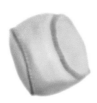

Small soft weighted ball

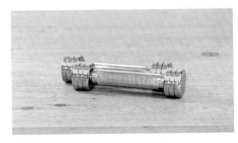

Hand weights (1 to 4 pounds)

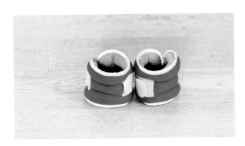

Ankle weights (1 to 1.5 pounds)

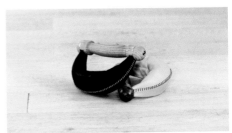

Swing weights

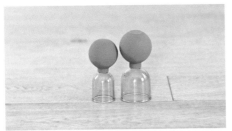

Cupping suction glass (35 or 50 mm diameter)

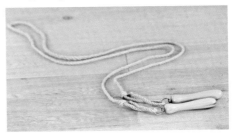

Jump rope

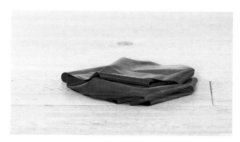

Resistance band

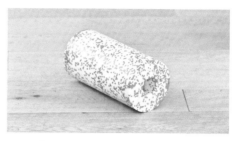

Large foam roller with smooth surface

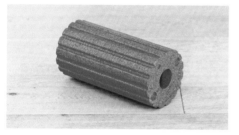

Large foam roller with corrugated surface

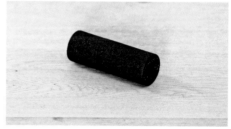

Mini foam roller

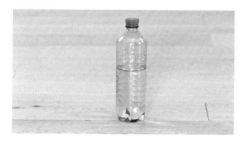

Half-full water bottle

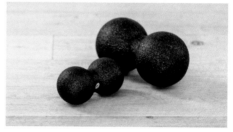

Large and small Duoball

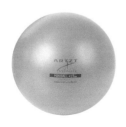

Overball

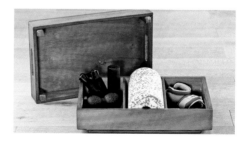

Fascia box with training tools

Basics of Fascia Training

Fascia training can be divided into four categories: elastic rebounding, fascial release, sensory refinement, and fascial stretching. Each category focuses on one of the collagen network's prominent characteristics. The goal of the training is to increase connective tissue resilience so it will become more elastic and tensile and therefore better able to withstand stress and strain.

Dynamic resistance

Kangaroos can jump much farther than could be explained strictly by the contractile force of their leg muscles. Upon closer analysis, scientists discovered and documented the so-called catapult mechanism. Here the tendons and fascia of the legs are preloaded like rubber bands and their targeted release then facilitates impressive jumps of up to 42 feet.

With the use of modern portable ultrasonic devices it has finally become possible in the last few years document a similar, highly efficient catapult effect in the human Achilles tendon. Even more surprising was the discovery that the human tissues showed the same impressive gazelle-like elastic storage capacity. This finding largely relates to the enormous storage capacity of the Achilles tendon, but we assume that, for instance, the strong sinewy fascia of the shoulder girdle or the back fascia possess similar kangaroo-like properties. In fascia training, we strengthen the catapult effect with a

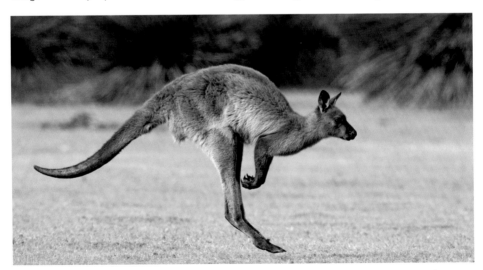

Vertical leap with catapult effect: With each jump the kangaroo utilizes stored elastic energy by preloading its strong Achilles tendons.

number of dynamic resistance exercises. The goal is to increase the storage capacity and elasticity of collagen fibers and thereby achieve healthy and vital resilience. Our first basic exercise, the flying sword, works, among other things, the thoracolumbar fascia. Flying sword is a powerful elastic rebound exercise designed for fostering a healthy and happy back.

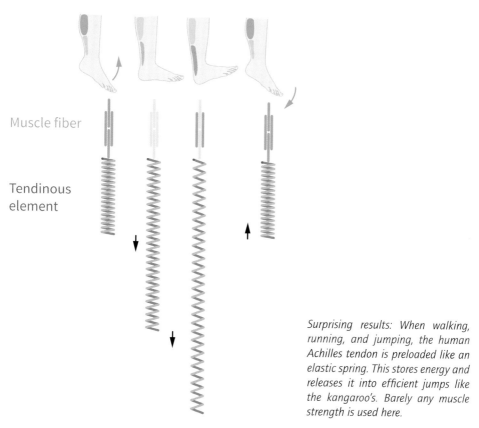

Muscle fiber

Tendinous element

Surprising results: When walking, running, and jumping, the human Achilles tendon is preloaded like an elastic spring. This stores energy and releases it into efficient jumps like the kangaroo's. Barely any muscle strength is used here.

Basic elastic rebound exercise: the flying sword

Tool: swing dumbbell or regular dumbbell

The flying sword is a powerful dynamic exercise that strengthens the elasticity of the front and back lines. For a true Viking type, this exercise is a blessing as long as it is done correctly.

Since this is a strengthening and athletic exercise performed with a long lever, it is contraindicated for people with acute back problems or instability of the lumbar spine or hip joints. If this is the case, you can complete exercises from the practice section on toning the connective tissue. There you will find a selection of appropriate strengthening exercises.

1. Stand with your feet hip-width apart, knees slightly bent, and the pelvis tilted forward slightly. Hold the weight with both hands and raise it above your head. Next make a slight whip-like motion as you bring the weight backward. Please note: As you swing the weight backward you must stabilize your lumbar spine by tightening your lower abdomen as though you were trying to pull it toward your lumbar spine. By doing so, you activate the fascial connection of the deep abdominal muscles with the thoracolumbar fascia. During the swinging motion the shoulder blades remain low and the thoracic spine should lengthen and extend backward like an elastic bamboo stalk to preload the fascia. This is the energy storage phase.

2. Once you have found a swinging rhythm, you can unload the fascia during the next step. Here the sternum pulls the upper body forward with a brief impulse and thereby initiates the forward and downward swinging motion. Vigorously guide the weight between your legs; the head follows, and in the final position the arms are fully extended to the back and upward. Now the back line is loaded during this preloaded position. Use this final position as the point of return and swing back to the starting position.

Variation for downward swing:

3. As you swing the weight downward, guide it past your body to the right and back, and then back up over your head, and with the next downward swing guide it past your body to the left and back. Actively involve the upper body and head in the side, down, and backward movement. Shift your weight to the leg on the side of the downward swing and bend that knee. These twists load and strengthen the lateral structures of the thoracolumbar fascia.

Variation for upward swing:

4. On the upward swing, swing the weight to the right and then back down between the legs. Next swing the weight up into the neutral overhead position, and back down between the legs, and finally with the next upward swing, swing the weight to the left and up.

If you are new to fascia training, five repetitions of the basic exercise are sufficient.

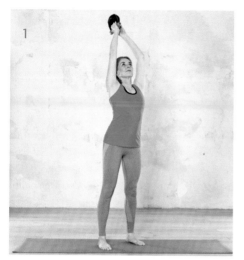
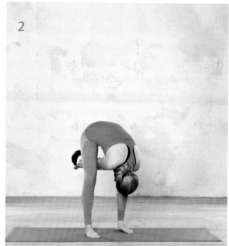
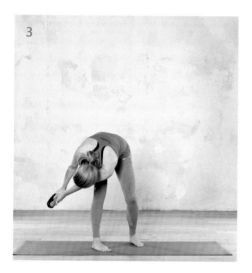
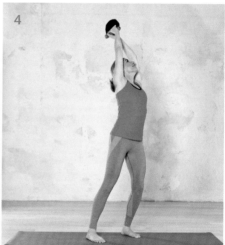

Fascial release

We already thoroughly covered self-treatment with the foam roller in the section "Rolling for rehydration" on page 54. Next we will discuss the practical application of fascial release and the slow fascial squeezing required for release and rehydration.

As previously mentioned, rolling does not only squeeze out accumulated tissue fluid but also has a refill effect since the moss-like fascial tissue subsequently becomes more water-binding. Fascia researchers found out that immediately after the fascial release, a kind of super compensation takes place and the fascia sponges then soaked up more water than before. Improved binding of water makes the fibers stiffer, more resilient, and firmer. A desirable effect, which we will build on with the following basic exercises.

The tools we will use in addition to the foam roller are different-sized balls to, for instance, roll out smaller areas like the plantar fascia.

Basic exercise for fascial release: rolling out the outer thigh

Tool: large foam roller with smooth surface

1. Lie on your left side propped on your left forearm with your elbow below your shoulder. Place the foam roller just below your left iliac crest; your left leg is extended, the right knee is bent, and the right foot is planted on the floor. You can place your free hand on the floor in front of your body for support. Now slowly roll the outer thigh from the iliac crest down towards the knee. As you move, imagine that the tissue is a sponge you are slowly squeezing with the pressure of the roller. Roll even slower in places that are particularly sensitive or painful and melt into the pressure.

2. As soon as the roller is just above the knee, slowly reverse and roll upward and back to the starting position. Stand up, take a few steps, and feel the difference from the other side.

You can repeat rolling one more time. Afterwards roll the outside of the right thigh.

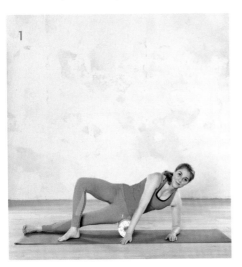
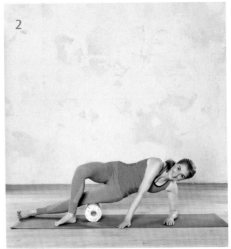

Sensory refinement

Whether we walk as gracefully as a queen or waddle like a duck, the question of how we move depends less on the genetic makeup with respect to motor abilities than on our self-awareness, proprioception. Surprisingly, this long-forgotten sixth sense is located in the fascial network. By now it is considered as proven that the fascia is equipped with numerous stretch receptors and sensitive nerves, and likely represent our largest sensory organ.

New is the finding that these sensory feelers reside primarily in the superficial layers of the fascia. Imagine the deep subcutaneous fascia sheath as a diving suit. This suit is covered with many small lights that light up like sensors with each movement and change in tension. The more detailed the stretch impulses, the more lights turn on inside and we are aware of every body movement, but this sensory refinement must be practiced and refined. It allows us to move through life with a supple elegance and a sense of well-being. In addition, an alert body sense is the best preventative of (back) pain. Pain researchers were able to prove that there is a definite gap between the sensory precision of people with healthy backs and those with back problems. When a chronic back pain patient is touched at a pressure point in the area of pain, he is unable to accurately localize the point of contact. His body-awareness lens has been dulled so much that when asked, he has a deviation of 2.5 to 3 inches from the actual point of contact. In people with healthy backs that deviation lies at approximately 1.5 inches. On the flip side, refining body awareness can ease myofascial pain.

Basic sensory refinement exercise: the spinal chain

1. In a standing position, bend your upper body forward and slightly bend your knees. Your feet are farther than hip-width apart and are firmly planted on the floor. Your body weight is evenly distributed between the three points of big toe, small toes, and heel. Keep your pelvis and head in alignment with your spine and brace your hands on your thighs. Pull your shoulder blades down and open the chest.

2 and 3. Now try to be aware of the individual thoracic vertebrae during small back-and-forth movements between the shoulder blades, pendular side-to-side movements, and finally figure eights in all directions. Take more time with spinal segments that move jerkily, and gradually the movements will flow smoothly. Let go of the idea that the spine is a rigid pillar where vertebrae have been firmly nailed on top of each other. Discover the movement of individual vertebrae as though they were strung on an elastic strand of pearls. The mental image and refined quality of movement will help you stimulate the body sense that resides within the fascial tissue.

Take a moment to notice the effects. Most likely your back will feel more agile and pleasantly invigorated in the areas you moved.

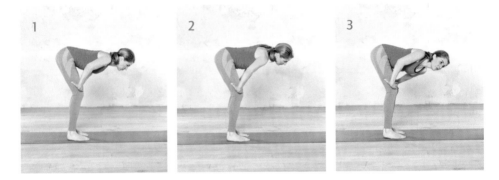

Variation: cobra spine

1. Start out on all fours. Now straighten your knees while lifting your sit bones toward the ceiling and pressing your heels towards the floor. At the same time, extend your arms forward and firmly plant your hands on the floor. The head is between the shoulders as an extension of the spine. Here the spinal chain is being pleasantly stretched in both directions and decompressed.

2. Now stimulate the movement of individual vertebrae via figure eights and micro movements. This releases restrictive tension in a stiff spine, letting it gradually turn into a snake-like spine: strong and flexible.

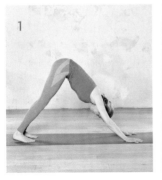 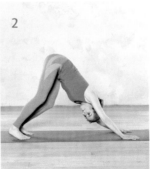 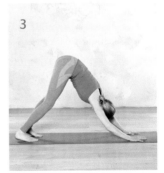

Fascial stretching

Cats don't have to learn how to stretch. They are by nature the world champions of stretching; they instinctively bend and stretch luxuriously in every direction. Stretching in every direction lubricates the fascia layers and facilitates coordinated movement. A cat stretches with abandon from its front paws to its back paws and in doing so, intuitively stretches long fascial chains and membranes that are linked over long distances.

But cats can teach us still more about stretching. Cats always look for new angles within the long-chain stretches and stretch in different directions. We use yet another cat stretch element during fascial stretching: the actively loaded stretch. Every cat owner's horror is when their four-legged darling digs its claws into the new leather sofa for a long and active stretch. Unlike the melting stretch, here the muscles are not relaxed but rather shortened. The contracted muscles load the stretch.

The be-all and end-all of fascial stretching

1. The longer the myofascial chain, the better. Choose stretch positions that involve multiple joints.

2. Vary directions and different angles within the stretch position in order to activate the three-dimensional fascia network in as many directions as possible.

3. Do passive, melting stretches with relaxed muscles. To do so, you relax (melt) into the stretch positions.

4. Include actively loaded stretches. Mini bounces, stretching against resistance, or using weights can activate the muscles within the long stretch position.

Basic fascial stretch: cat

1. Stand facing a chair with your knees slightly bent and your feet hip-width apart. Bend over with your arms extended and your hands resting on the seat of the chair. Hands are shoulder-width apart and hips are stacked over heels. The head is an extension of the spine. As you do so, imagine the crown of your head reaching forward.

2. Feel your sit bones. Now push your right sit bone back and upward while straightening the right knee and bending the left knee. At the same time, spread the fingers of your left hand, open the palm, and stretch the fingers forward and up as though you were extending your claws.

As a melting stretch, hold this position for one minute. As an actively loaded stretch, do mini bounces originating in the feet and into the superficial back line. Stretch your leg with 3, 5, 7, or 10 mini bounces and switch sides.

3. Now return to the starting position, push both sit bones back and up, and straighten your legs. Lift your heels off the floor, round your lower back, and stretch the superficial back line with a long cat back arch. Return to the starting position with a slow, smooth movement.

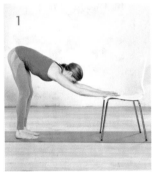 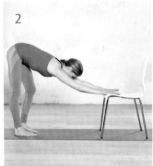 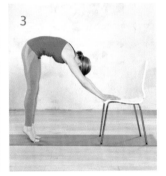

Forbidden mini bounces

For years we have banished bouncing from our repertoire as a no-go. In fascia training we dust off this form of bouncing and practice mini bounces. Here the emphasis lies on *mini*. This bouncing movement comprises a radius of 1 to 2 inches, meaning it is small and controlled. We definitely don't want you to forcefully pull on your tissue with uncontrolled movements. That would make the bouncing ban appropriate because it would result in pulled muscles or injuries.

Viking and Temple Dancer Dos and Don'ts

For stiff Viking types, actively loaded stretches are a good way to effectively increase flexibility, but since this book focuses primarily on soft connective tissue types (i.e., hypermobile temple dancers), Viking types will not find a specific exercise program here that will increase flexibility.

If you are a rather stiff type or have individual shortened fascia chains, you can certainly do the exercise program that tightens connective tissue, but you should always stretch out the chain you worked at the end of the exercise sequence. To do so, return to the position of the first exercise to refine the respective chain. All of these are terminal stretch positions that are perfect for the subsequent long stretches. To finish, we especially recommend the melting stretch. Hold this position for 1 to 2 minutes and take soft and melting breaths into the respective stretch.

If you would like to work more extensively on your flexibility, you can find recommendations for physical therapists and trainers under "Tools and Tips" on page 176.

However, terminal stretches that focus on additional lengthening—whether melting or actively loaded—are not suitable for hypermobile connective tissue types. This next segment offers specific power principles for toning connective tissue in temple dancer types.

The Success Formula for Healthy and Firm Connective Tissue

Most likely you are now eagerly anticipating the exercises that tighten the connective tissue. In this particular training, we will focus on three of the described basic principles: sensory refinement, elastic rebound, and hydrating regeneration via fascial release self-treatment. Finally, the fourth building block—a new, specific toning power principle that replaces fascial stretches—makes training particularly efficient.

Power principle to tighten the collagen sheath surrounding muscle

With our power principle, the muscle is loaded in the area where the working muscle fibers are shortened the most. For instance, in the biceps the toning position (i.e., to increase muscle tension) would be maximum elbow flexion. Here the transverse collagen fibers running along the muscle belly are maximally loaded. This is readily identifiable by the bulging muscle belly. In this position you load the muscle by adding highly dosed impulses via bouncing movements. The intention is to aggravate the fibroblasts to the point of rousing them from their metabolic comfort zone so they will create more collagen over the next two to three days, particularly in the muscle belly's transverse fascia sheath. On the other hand, for the triceps the respective position in which the working fibers are shortened the most and the muscle belly is most bulbous is a nearly straight elbow. Anyone who abhors arm flab at the triceps should work them with deliberate mini bounces with nearly straight elbows (see photo).

In addition we try to exhaust the muscle fibers in this maximally shortened position based on the justified assumption that the tissue will be restructured in the coming weeks and as a result the muscle's working range will shift towards the short area. Usually the working range lies halfway between maximal stretch and maximal shortening. In other words, it is a way to also tighten the muscle while shortening it.

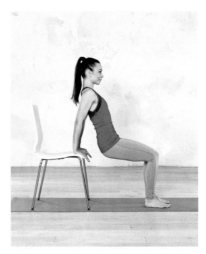

The success formula

Refine + bounce + tone + regenerate = Tighten the connective tissue

---

How do I build a healthy and firm connective tissue body?

These are most certainly questions you are interested in: How long does it take for the collagen network to regenerate? How often do I have to work out and at what intensity?

Here are the three golden rules for fascia training.

Training recommendation 1: the patience of a bamboo gardener

We like to compare the collagen network to a brittle bamboo hut that must be restored with fresh, juicy reeds. Muscle size can be increased within three months. Collagen regeneration takes longer. Researchers assume that collagen formation takes place anywhere from 3 to 6 months. In my experience, there is a noticeable increase in elasticity and tonicity after three months of regular fascia training. One positive of the sustained collagen formation is the resulting major sustainability.

For instance, while muscle quickly breaks down during an illness, the elastic bamboo hut remains. Cultivate the patience of a bamboo gardener! He waters the bamboo seeds for months without a visible sign of growth. After tireless care the new shoot emerges and quickly grows to the sky, and as it does so it surpasses all the other plants of the forest in height and elasticity.

Training recommendation 2: the toggle-switch principle

Muscles are more like dimmers; the fascia is more like a toggle switch. Studies done with older women show that muscles registered definite growth even with moderate strength training at one third of maximum strength, but that has no effect on tendons and other fascia with dense parallel fibers such as aponeuroses. Only at 70% of maximum strength did a growth impulse in tendons and aponeuroses occur. It is different with intramuscular connective tissue. Here approximately 30% of maximum strength is enough to stimulate collagen formation.

Hence we can deduce the following training recommendation: The strong, parallel fiber structures like tendons and aponeuroses are more like stiff toggle switches that require an intensive training impulse. The more delicate intramuscular connective tissue and the lattice-like muscle sheath require only a moderate training impulse. With respect to repetitions, a recently published study by Danish researcher Michael Kjær showed that an intensive training impulse is achieved after just a few dozen repetitions. It doesn't make much sense to do additional repetitions after that, based on the motto: More is better. For this reason we recommend to start with 5, 7, or 10 repetitions when training with rebound elasticity, and to increase them carefully and by a few repetitions over time. This will prevent overload damage from too many repetitions while still stimulating increased collagen production in tendons and aponeuroses.

Since muscular toning is a specific variation of fascia training to tighten connective tissue, it is important to max out repetitions until muscle exhaustion during these training units. Here the muscle is deliberately loaded in the short range. The result is that it permanently shortens its working range, particularly at the center and length of the muscle. The desired side effect is the strengthening and tightening of the myofascial tissue.

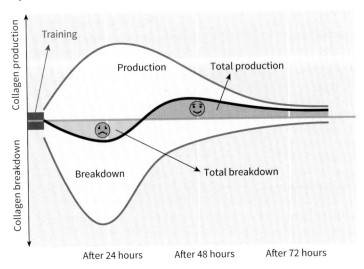

Fibroblasts initially react to the training impulse with an increased breakdown of collagen. Only after 24 to 48 hours is collagen production, meaning the synthesis of fresh fibers, back in the plus. Conclusion: If you want to build a healthy fascia within 6 to 12 months, you should work them two to three times a week while allowing the collagen tissue to regenerate in between workouts.

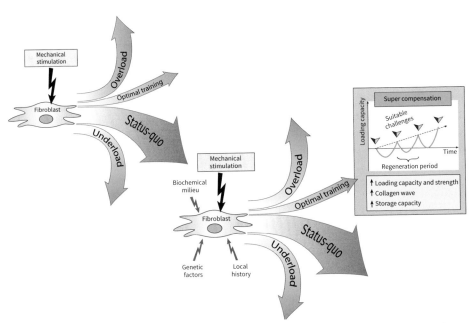

Underloading is just as bad as overloading. The connective tissue architects, the fibroblasts, require intensive but suitable mechanical stimulation. Here factors such as individual history, genetic predisposition, and internal biochemical milieu play an important role for an optimal outcome.

Training recommendation 3: respect the regeneration period

The good thing about fascia training is that you will make great gains with short and intensive training units. One intensive training unit two to three times a week is sufficient, but you should definitely wait 48 to 72 hours before adding the next training impulse. As you can see on the left side of the above illustration, a training impulse initiates collagen production, but collagen breakdown increases at the same time. This is absolutely a desirable process to dismantle the brittle hut, but only after 48 to 72 hours does collagen production predominate. In the meantime, let the myofibroblasts do their work and don't add any additional active dynamic impulses such as elastic rebound and muscle toning. During the following weeks, more fresh collagen will be collected and you will achieve your goal—toning your connective tissue.

The Basic Positions

Before you begin with the training, we will show you all of the basic positions you will need to complete the different exercises via the following outline.

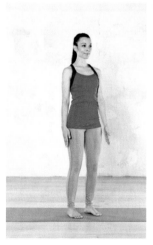

Tightening the catsuit

In the starting position, stand tall with your feet parallel and hip-width apart.

Tighten your plantar fascia: Tighten your large toe, small toes, and the outside edge of your foot all the way to the heel. In this three-point stance, actively press your feet into the floor. As you do so, imagine trying to leave a visible footprint in the dirt.

Tighten your fingertips: Imagine trying to pull each fingertip down towards the floor. Tighten your fascial chains all the way to the shoulders and pull the shoulders down as well. This slight preloading, which you should hold during your bouncing exercises, is absolutely sufficient but also necessary to optimize elastic strengthening.

Lengthening the crown of the head (galea aponeurotica): Gently lengthen your neck as though you were trying to reach the ceiling or the sky with the crown of your head. Notice how the neck fascia prestretches and the cervical spine elongates.

Activating the fascial corset

In a standing position, slightly bend your knees and rest your hands on the front of your thighs. Keep your back straight by reaching forward and up with the crown of the head and back and down with your sit bones. Now try to pull your lower abdomen towards your lumbar spine. Please do not use maximal tension but rather imagine that you are trying to stretch a piece of plastic foil from your lower abdomen to your lumbar vertebrae. This flattens the stomach and stabilizes the low back via the cross-linking of the deep abdominal muscles' collagen structures to the thoracolumbar fascia.

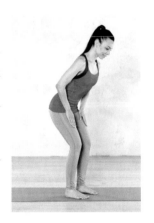

All-fours position

Begin on all fours with your wrists below your shoulders and your knees below your hips. Hands are firmly planted on the floor and fingers are slightly spread. Now pull your shoulders out slightly and squeeze your shoulder blades together so your chest opens towards the floor. Stabilize the lumbar spine by pulling the lower abdomen

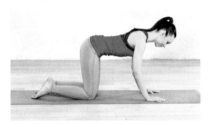

towards the lumbar spine (i.e., activating the fascial corset). In the basic position the back should be long and straight from the crown of the head to the sit bones.

The squat

Stand with your feet hip-width apart and bend your knees. Rest your hands palm-down against the front of your thighs. Keep your back straight by reaching forward and up with the crown of the head and back and down with your sit bones. In a squat your legs are parallel and your bodyweight is shifted to the outside of your feet and heels.

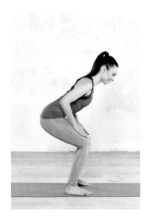

The lunge

Take a big step into a forward lunge. As you do so, bend the forward knee and support yourself on your forward thigh with both arms. Knees, calves, and foot form a vertical line. The back leg is extended, and the heel and outside edge of the foot press firmly into the floor so that the fascia surrounding the ankle is activated and stable. In this position the back, spine, and head form a straight line.

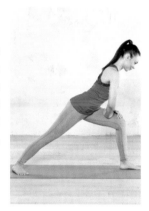

Forearm plank

Lie on your stomach, resting on your forearms. The elbows are below the shoulders. Pull your shoulder blades down while reaching up with the crown of the head. Legs and toes are extended.

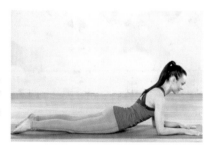

Lateral reclining position

Lie on your side and extend legs and toes as an extension of the upper body. Your upper arm rests loosely on your side, the lower arm is extended and supports your head. In this position, activate the abdominal muscles to slightly pull your waist away from the floor.

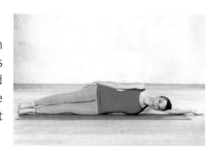

Side plank

Lie on your side with your legs extended and your feet flexed. Now lift your upper body off the floor by propping yourself up on your forearm. The elbow is below the shoulder. Next tighten your muscles to also lift the pelvis off the floor. You can support yourself with your free hand in front of your body or let the hand rest on your hip. In the plank position the body forms a straight line from head to toe.

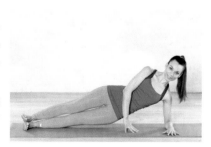

Training Recommendations for Practice

The elastic rebound and toning elements denote the dynamic and strengthening exercises. You may be surprised how demanding these exercises are at the beginning of the training program.

In the beginning 3, 5, 7, or 10 bouncing repetitions can be totally sufficient. Here it is important that you know and respect your personal limit. Each week add 1 to 2 repetitions, but avoid overloading with too many repetitions, especially when doing jumps.

However, for the toning exercises to be successful, it is essential that you come up against your personal exhaustion limit.

To work on some particularly important body regions such as, for instance, tightening the thighs, you can choose from several exercises. In the beginning it is sufficient to complete one exercise from each category of the success formula sequence: refine, bounce, tone, regenerate. To avoid monotony over time, frequently build another exercise into your program. Once you have reached 20 or more repetitions per exercise, we recommend combining two exercises for that same area so you can reach the necessary intensity. For example, when toning the thighs: for the first round do the easy thigh-tightening exercise without weight followed by the advanced thigh-tightening exercise with ankle weight or the advanced thigh-tightening exercise with resistance band.

The refining training element requires a different approach. Here the focus is on sensory awareness. For hypermobile people of the temple dancer type, this is an important health-maintaining topic. Their detailed perception is nearly *body blind*, particularly with respect to terminal stretching. Due to their excessive flexibility, they stretch beyond the healthy limits, meaning they do not *hear* the groaning "Stop!" of their joints. The danger: Over the years their joints come apart at the seams.

So when doing the refining exercises the motto is not "More is better." Instead the focus should be on quality of movement as well as feeling or listening to the body: How does this movement feel? It is important to notice at which point there is a lack of precision of movement control and accuracy of perception. Here temple dancer types should actively work on detailed movements and graduated angle changes and bring this area back to a state of alert body awareness. At the end of the refining exercises, take a moment to notice how you feel. After that your proprioception, meaning your sense of movement that resides primarily in the fascia, is switched on. Then you will be on the safe side with your dynamic strengthening exercises and can properly control them and perform them correctly.

Foam rollers and cupping glasses are used to regenerate the connective tissue. When working with the foam roller, we use two different applications with different effects.

First comes the invigorating and toning rolling. Here you roll back and forth five or six times with considerable pressure along the respective fascia.

Second is the slow and rehydrating rolling. Here it is important to push the fluids through the tissue in many different directions with a slow and continuous rolling movement. One round is sufficient here. A second rolling or massage will intensify the effect, but should also be done slowly and thoroughly. A slow and thorough application is more beneficial than two or more quick, short rounds.

Shoulder-Elbow Chain

Shapely upper arms and shoulders are a lovely sight. But since we rarely work hand-over-hand at the office or run across the street on all fours, our arms often get unshapely and flabby. But it doesn't have to be that way!

In this segment you will find a number of effective exercises to strengthen the upper arms over all. We also specifically target the deltoid, which you might be familiar with from the impressive upper-arm contour of many celebrities, most of all Michelle Obama. Her strong and shapely upper arms regularly make the headlines. You, too, can have such a defined contour, and here are the exercises to get you there. The nice thing is that toned muscles don't just look good, but they feel good, too. Shoulder movement is smoother and arms move with powerful suppleness.

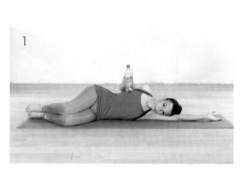

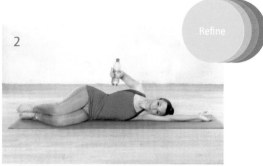

Refine

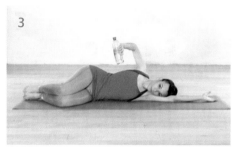

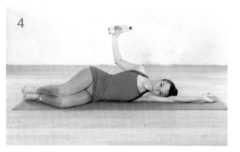

Fish fin

Tool: a half-full water bottle

1. Lie on your left side and bend your knees. The left arm is extended and supports the head. The right hand holds the water bottle. Bend the right elbow and pull it back.

2, 3 and 4. Now move your right arm to the side and overhead at different angles and in different directions much like a fish's fin, meaning in a fluid motion. The movement of the water in the bottle continuously creates moments of surprising stimulation that will challenge you to refine your coordination. A brief moment of checking in to see how you feel is well worth it. You will probably feel a distinct difference between the moving side and the still side. Next switch to the right side and repeat the exercise with your left arm.

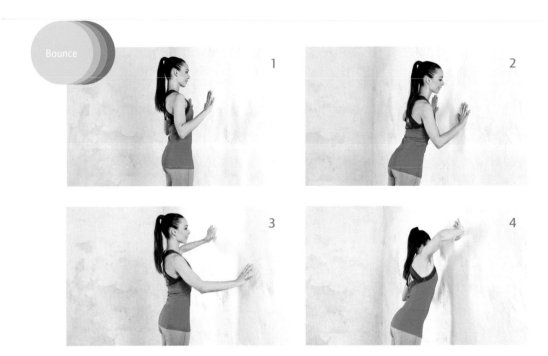

Power arms

1 and 2. Stand about three feet away from a wall with your legs hip-width apart. Tighten your catsuit and then bend your elbows with your palms facing the wall. Now let yourself fall forward and then bounce back off the wall like a rubber ball.

3 and 4. Next add the lateral movements to load your collagen sheath in as many areas as possible. To do so, plant your hands in different positions and alternate bouncing more to the left and to the right, and then back to the center.

Do 3, 5, 7, or 10 repetitions per variation; slowly increase.

Please note: Always maintain the tension in your longitudinal axis, from your feet to the crown of the head. This will also help keep you from arching your back. It is important to keep continuous basic tension in the arms so they can push off the wall and bounce back after a brief contact with the wall.

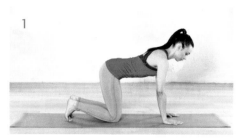
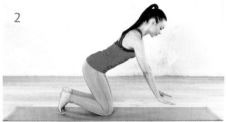
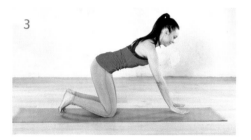
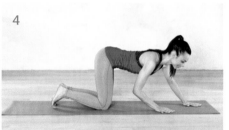
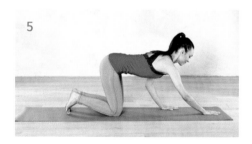

Power arms on the floor

1. Get down on all fours. Shift your bodyweight forward until your chest opens but your shoulders remain stable.

2 and 3. Now briefly push off with your arms and then gently and softly catch your body weight again with your hands.

4 and 5. Now plant your hands on the floor in different positions. Alternate bouncing more to the right and to the left, and back to the center.

Do 3, 5, 7, or 10 repetitions per variation; slowly increase.

Please note: Maintain body tension particularly in the chest and shoulder areas and keep the contact between hands and floor brief.

Tip for even more power

You an increase the tension in the arm fascia by, for instance, doing the power arms exercise on a windowsill later.

Tone

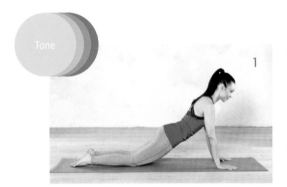

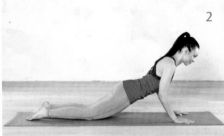

Triceps tightener

1. Start in a forearm plank and plant the hands below the shoulders and extend the arms to push up into a supported plank. Open the chest and reach up with the crown of the head. The pelvis is slightly raised and the tops of the feet rest on the floor.

2. Now firmly press your hands into the floor and bob up and down with the arms whereby the elbows bend very little and never fully extend. Your bounces should be quick, small, and dynamic.

The progression of this exercise is the following reverse plank dip on a chair.

Work your muscles to the point of muscle exhaustion.

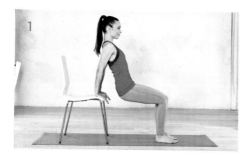
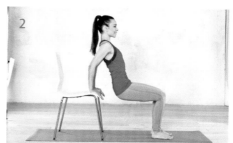
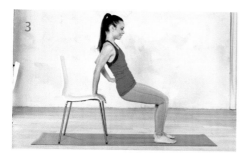
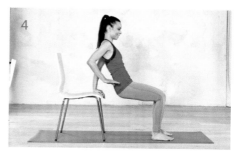

Reverse-plank dip on a chair

1. Support yourself on the seat of a chair as shown in the photo. Firmly press your palms into the seat, rotate and open your collarbones slightly to the outside, and pull the shoulders down. Your feet steadily press firmly against the floor and the crown of the head reaches towards the ceiling.

2. Maintain body tension and start to slightly bend your elbows and straighten them again to create impulses with these mini bounces.

3 and 4. To intensify this exercise, shift your bodyweight to the right arm and bounce while removing the left arm from the seat. Then shift the weight to the left arm and remove the right arm from the seat.

Work until you have exhausted the muscles.

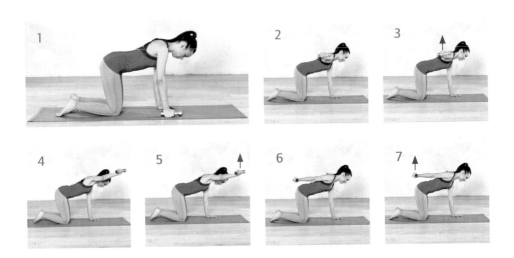

Deltoid tightener

Tool: hand weight

1. Start on all fours and plant your hands below the shoulders and your knees below the hips. Hold the weight in your right hand. The back is straight and stays that way during the entire exercise.

2 and 3. Maintain the muscle tension of your starting position. Extend the right arm to the side and make little bouncing up-and-down movements.

4, 5, 6, and 7. Now bounce your arm from the side position to the front, back to the side, and finally to the back. The arm remains fully extended during all of the bouncing movements. Now bounce back to the starting position and then work the other arm.

Work each side until you have exhausted the muscles.

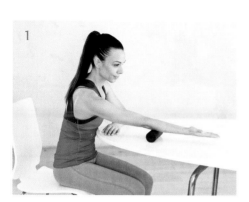 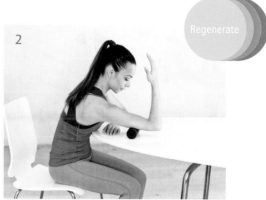

Regenerate

Rolling the arm

Tool: mini foam roller

1. Sit on a chair with your back straight and rest your extended right arm on the table. Place the mini foam roller under your forearm with the palm facing the ceiling. Now roll your arm vigorously and languorously.

2. Bend the elbow so the palm faces your face. Place the mini foam roller under your upper arm and roll it vigorously and languorously. Next repeat with the left arm.

Everyday exercise: the purse lift

Don't carry your purse with your arms hanging down, but rather raise your arms laterally. First pull the shoulders down before laterally raising your arm along with your purse. Hold this position for as long as possible, but at least for 30 seconds. Then switch sides. After a short break, repeat the exercise for a second time.

Chest-Biceps Chain

The following exercises focus primarily on fascia training for the biceps because not only does this muscle shape the upper arm, it also interconnects with the chest muscles' collagen sheath and therefore affects the tightening of the chest.

Sitting still for long periods of time and weight fluctuations or hormonal influences can cause the breasts to sag, and if nothing else, aging affects the firmness of breast tissue. Of course there are push-up bras that cleverly hide the toll gravity takes. Nevertheless, by doing specific fascia exercises women can strengthen the tension of the collagen network and activate the body's own collagen wonder bra.

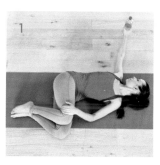 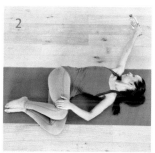 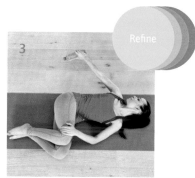

Refine

Chest opener

Tool: a half-full water bottle

1. Lie on your left side and bend both knees. Hold the water bottle in your right hand and rest the extended right arm sideways on the floor. Turn your head to the right so you can see your hand. To stabilize the position, hold on to your right thigh with your left hand. If you are a contortionist, you can probably easily rest the entire right arm on the floor and the chest opens slightly into this twist.

2 and 3. Lift your right arm a couple inches off the floor and now play with fluid angle changes. To do so, move the arm toward the head in a slow fluid motion, and then back to the starting position at the side, and then down toward the pelvis. If your arm drops to the floor in some places, seemingly on its own, those are areas that lack perception and where you will need to control your coordination deliberately and with precision.

If you are more of a Viking type, your arm probably hangs in the air. Stop at those places where the tension is particularly intense to even slightly painful, and melt into the stretch for 1 to 2 minutes. To dissolve adhesions, choose multiple positions, some closer to the pelvis and some closer to the head. Then switch sides.

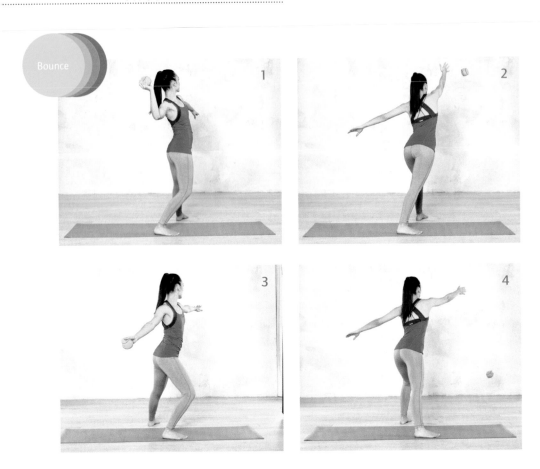

Bounce

Arm catapult

Tool: small weighted ball or ankle weight

1 and 2. Hold the ball in your right hand and stand with your legs astride with the left leg forward. Now reach way back with the hand holding the ball so that the fascia at the front of the body from the crown of the head to the toes is prestretched and the entire spine elongates. The upper body and thoracic spine should bend back like a reed in the wind, the sternum initiates the throwing motion, and the arm follows last with an energetic throw. In doing so, you load the fascia even more and utilize the arm catapult in the best possible way.

At the end of the throwing motion, remain in the stable stance. The weight is shifted to the forward foot, the upper body follows the forward arm movement and the fingers flex with the throw of the ball.

3 and 4. Now practice different ways of throwing to optimally activate the biceps chain. Throw the ball in the classic throwing position with an unloading backswing from above to the back, but also originating from below and from the back. Vary the throw several times. Next switch legs and complete the exercise with the left arm.

Do 3, 5, 7, or 10 repetitions per variation; increase slowly.

Tip for more dynamism

These exercises are dynamic because they focus on throwing. My studio has a designated throwing station and handmade leather balls (see "Tools and Tips" on page 176) that feel good in the hand and are easy to throw against the wall. If you have a suitable wall (be careful, my initial enthusiastic attempts resulted in plaster raining down) and a firm pillow or bolster, you can try the featured exercises at home. Otherwise look for a garage wall or get a TOGU medicine ball for throwing exercises with a bigger ball (e.g., see the power throw on page 123). These are cushioned balls of different weights used in fitness training, and they will be kinder to walls and neighbors.

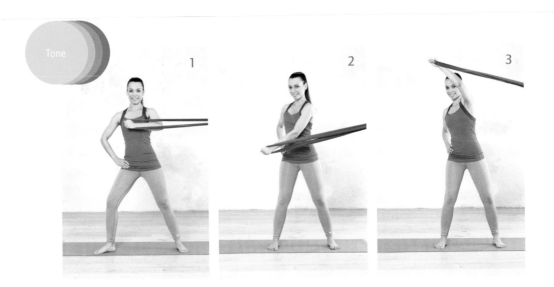

Chest tightener with resistance band

Tool: resistance band

A resistance band fastened to a door handle is a great and effective way to do your fascial fitness program at home.

1. Loop one end of the resistance band over a door handle. Hold the other end of the band in your left hand and take a few steps forward so the band has noticeable tension. Now stand in a wide straddle position parallel to your pulling direction. Make sure your stance is stable and tighten up your catsuit. Now lift your left arm to chest level, bend the elbow, and hold your forearm close to your chest. Rest your right hand on your hip. In this basic position, the resistance band is loaded.

2. From the basic position, pull the resistance band diagonally downward in front of your pelvis. In the final position the arm is fully extended and close to the body. Hold this position and boost the effect via mini bounces.

3. Return to the basic position and then pull the resistance band close to the chest, to the right and upward. Fully extend the arm, hold this final position and bounce. As a variation, incrementally bounce from one final position into the other. Switch sides and work the right arm.

Work each side until you have exhausted the muscles.

Tip for practicing at your fitness facility

Any of the exercises you do at home with the resistance band can also be done with the cable pull at your fitness facility. The cable pull is one of my favorite apparatuses for connective tissue strengthening. It allows you to set the optimal resistance and to gradually increase it.

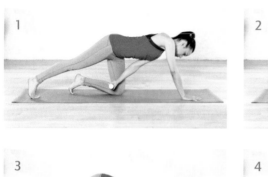
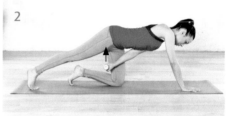
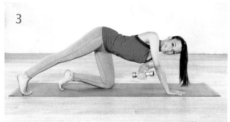
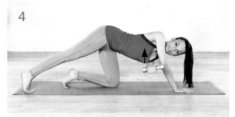

Chest tightener with hand weight

Tool: hand weight

(Suggestion: Start with 2 pounds of weight and increase the weight to 4 pounds over the coming weeks.)

1 and 2. Begin on all fours. Extend the right leg back, flex the foot, and tuck the toes of both feet. Hold the weight in your left hand, and extend the left arm to the back along the inside of the left leg. Bounce toward the ceiling.

3 and 4. Now incrementally bounce from the starting position to the side. In the final position your arm is extended forward at chest level and you continue to bounce toward the ceiling. Switch sides and work the right arm.

Work each side until you have exhausted the muscles.

Please note: To achieve the strengthening effect, it is important that the elbow be straight and the upper arm make small controlled bouncing motions into the tension of the chest muscle. Only then will you specifically reach the collagen structures. When bouncing, please make sure that you hold the extended arm close to the chest. Bounce with small controlled motions. Only then will you optimally stimulate the collagen structures of the sheath.

Connective tissue massage for the chest

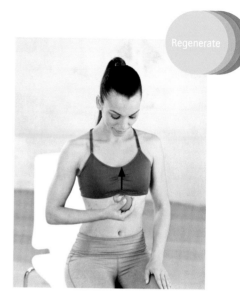

Tool: Cupping glass

During this exercise you will work directly on the skin. Spread a small amount of oil on your chest to facilitate continuous gliding. Pick up the cupping glass and trace two massage tracks:

1. Start the first track at the lower end of the sternum (the xiphisternum), make an arc to the right, and then move up to the armpit.

2. The second track moves from the xiphisternum in a straight line along the sternum and up to the collarbone, and then to the armpit. This specifically stimulates lymphatic drainage.

Everyday exercise: jungle gym

Find a playground near you and hang from the monkey bars or the climbing net with both arms. Swing a few times from one side to the other. Over the coming weeks, try to hold on with just one arm and swing to the other arm. The jungle gym is extremely challenging and super-effective for tightening arms and chest.

Abdominal Network: Straight, Oblique, and Transverse Abdominal Muscles

Here the focus is on your strong core, meaning a tight stomach and a slender waist. And here, too, this rule applies: Just building muscle mass doesn't give you that coveted hourglass figure. What matters is strengthening the collagen network surrounding the straight, oblique, and transverse abdominal muscles with toning exercises.

When this network is strong, it creates, among other things, stability, that flat tight lower abdomen and the definition of the classic six pack. Having washboard abs isn't just the professed goal of our training, but regaining a tight stomach after, for instance, a pregnancy or creating a shapely silhouette is definitely worth striving for. The good news: Our exercises make it possible!

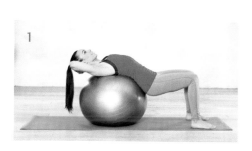
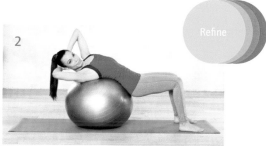

Refine

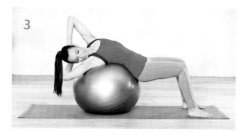
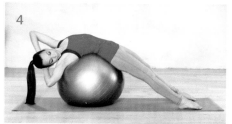

Activating the core network

Tool: stability ball

1. Lie with your back on a stability ball, plant your feet, and keep your knees parallel during the exercise. Cross the arms behind your head and support your neck with your hands. Now roll the ball from the shoulder blades down toward the pelvis and back up to the starting position.

2. Stretch the upper and lower abdominal areas and the obliques in different directions with a fluid motion.

3 and 4. As you do so, include the diagonal fascia chain by twisting the upper body to the right, then stretch out a little longer by reaching with the elbow and extending the legs. Return to the starting position, and then twist your upper body to the left to also work the other diagonal lengthwise.

All movements should be relaxed, smooth, and soothing.

Rules for stomach-tightening exercises

With all toning exercises:

- The lower abdominal area remains flat during the entire exercise.
- The upper body never drops below the starting position.
- The range of motion is no more than ¾ of an inch to 1 inch.
- Bounce until muscles are exhausted.

Power sounds

You have heard martial artists make power sounds. They are, for instance, the sounds of a karate master's exhale as he breaks a brick and accompanies that dynamic action with a brief, explosive "huh" or "heh."

The following exercise will include power sounds. The diaphragm activity causes the internal transverse abdominal muscles to contract, and by reflex the pelvic floor is engaged elastically.

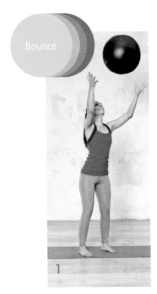
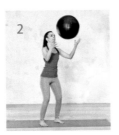
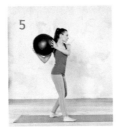
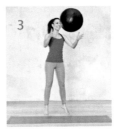
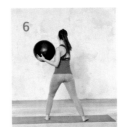
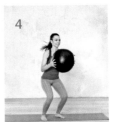
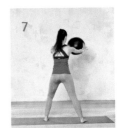

Bounce

Power throw

Tool: medicine ball or ATX CrossFit ball (or a firm pillow or bolster as an alternative)

We use throwing movements with both arms to tighten the core network and the body's fascial corset of the lower abdomen and pelvic floor. We additionally load these structures with the weight of the ball and increase their elastic resistance.

1 and 2. Throw the ball up into the air with both hands and catch it with elastic knees.

3 and 4. Jump into the air with both legs as you throw the ball up, and then catch it again with elastic knees.

5. Hold the ball in front of the body with both hands and stand a sufficient distance from a wall. Build up full-body tension for the throw. To do so, turn your upper body to the right and step back with your right foot, and then move the ball far to the back and side. Next. you hurl the ball forward against the wall. Repeat the exercise by opening your upper body up to the left. Accompany your dynamic throw with the power sound "huh" or "heh."

6 and 7. Stand facing the wall with your legs in a stable straddle position. Similar to a two-handed backhand in tennis, now turn only your upper body to the left and let both arms follow. Feet and knees remain parallel and point forward. Hurl the ball with an accompanying power sound. After the throw, remain in your position and maintain your full-body tension.

Do 3, 5, 7, or 10 repetitions per variation; gradually increase.

Tone

1

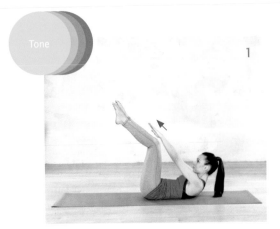

2

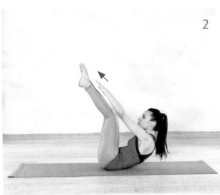

Tightening the straight abdominal muscle

1. Lie on your back and raise your lower legs slightly more than 90° relative to your upper legs, and point your toes. Now lift your head off the floor, leaving a hand's width of space between your chin and your chest, and tighten your lower abdomen. Now extend both arms to the ceiling to activate the lower part of the straight abdominal muscle. Hold this position for a moment and bounce with your fingertips toward your toes.

2. You work the upper part of the straight abdominal muscle by lifting your upper body a little higher and widening the knee angle. Hold this position and bounce with your fingertips toward your toes.

Finally, vigorously bounce from the position of the first exercise into the higher position and back down to the starting position.

Finish by resting your arms and legs on the floor and stretching out long.

Continue the exercise until you have exhausted the muscles.

Tightening the obliques

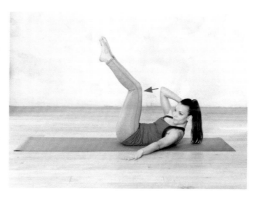

Lie on your back and raise your lower legs slightly more than 90° relative to your upper legs and point your toes. Lift your head off the floor, leaving a hand's width of space between your chin and your chest, and tighten your lower abdomen. Extend your left arm on the floor alongside your body and place your right hand at the back of your head. Now bounce with your right elbow towards your left knee without pulling the elbow forward; the movement originates in the belly. Switch sides through the center.

Work each side until you have exhausted the muscles.

Please note: Move your legs far enough away from your upper body to activate the lower abdomen while still keeping it flat during the entire exercise. If the lower abdomen begins to bulge during the bouncing phase, move your knees closer to your upper body again. Otherwise you will stress the lumbar spine and the pelvic floor.

Tightening all of the abdominal muscles

You can tighten all of the abdominal muscles with a power combination. Begin with the exercise targeting the lower part of the straight abdominal muscle and then continue directly to the oblique abdominals. Then return to the center and immediately move on to working the upper part of the straight abdominal. Finish by bouncing from the top position down to the starting position. Now you can rest your head and stretch out.

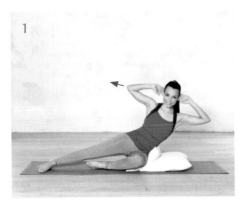 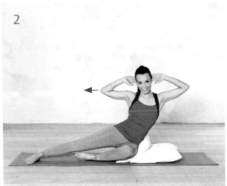

Tightening the waist (advanced)

1. Sit on your left side and bend the left knee in front of your body; keep the right leg extended. You can support your pelvis with a pillow as shown in the photo. Hold your hands at the back of the head; elbows point to the outside. Now tighten the muscles in your upper body all the way to the top of the head and reach upward with the crown. As you do so, imagine that you are trying to touch your right foot with your right elbow. Hold the high position and do small bouncing waist-bends.

2. Finally pull the upper body a little higher and intensify the exercise with quick and firm mini bounces.

Please note: Even if it is strenuous, the range of motion for the mini bounces is 1 to 2 inches!

Next change your sitting position and work the other side of the waist.

Work each side until you have exhausted the muscles.

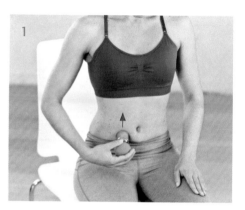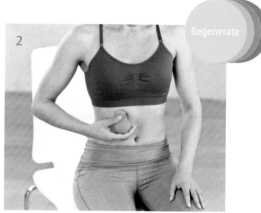

Abdominal connective tissue massage

Tool: Cupping glass

This massage to tighten abdominal connective tissue can be done on the entire stomach.

1 and 2. To tone the tissue, vigorously pull the tool across the entire stomach at a brisk pace from the bottom to the top. Make sure the skin is lifted away from the subcutaneous fatty tissue and maintain a steady pushing motion. Use a little massage oil if needed.

Please note: If you have a scar on your stomach, you need to proceed differently and more gently. Reduce the pace to super-slow. We suggest 1/3 of an inch for each breathing cycle. Since scars are often linked to pronounced adhesions below the skin that can sometimes cause discomfort or pain, we try to release them with the slower pace. The goal is to allow the individual skin and tissue layers to once again move freely past each other. For pronounced adhesions, we recommend treatment by a chiropractor trained in myofascial release such as a DO or Rolfer with the expertise to release these adherences (you can find suggestions under "Tools and Tips" on page 176).

Diagonal Lat-Glutes Muscle Chain

This segment is all about a healthy back and the diagonal chain that provides an elastic connection between the upper body and lower body. The thoracolumbar fascia plays an important part here together with the gluteus maximus via elastic collagenous connections.

The following exercises focus on a back that is designed for loading and physical demands, and its perfectly structured extension that is limited to Homo sapiens, the buttocks. None of our related primates have such an attractive backside as we do. Such a biological legacy obligates, and it is well worth working this fascia twice a week for a happy and healthy back.

1

2

Refine

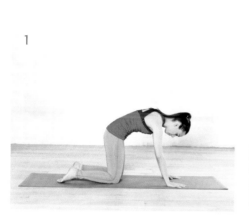

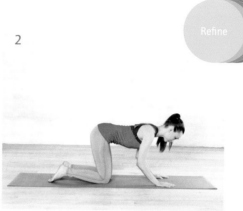

Cat stretches

1. On all fours, stretch your back by rounding it into a big cat back arch. The head is forward and down, the sit bones pull back and down. Hold this flexed position and stretch in all directions like a cat. As you do so, you stretch the thoracolumbar fascia in different lateral and diagonal directions and changing angles.

2. Alternate between a cat back arch and a straight back. Elongate your sit bones into the back as an extension of the spine and pull the crown of the head forward. Pull the shoulder blades together and open the chest. Then move back into the long cat back arch.

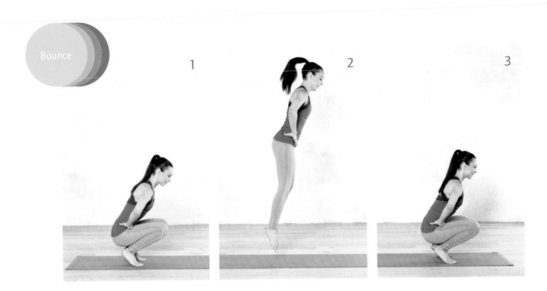

Bounce

1   2   3

Frog jump

1. Start in a low and wide squat with your feet slightly wider than hip-width apart. Shift your weight forward to the front of the feet and rest your hands on your hips.

2 and 3. Leap up and then land back in a deep squat. Work quickly, dynamically, and vigorously, and use only your legs without help from your arms.

Do 3, 5, 7, or 10 repetitions; gradually increase.

Everyday exercise: African lift

Lift a bag positioned at your side (no more than 13 pounds) with both hands. Do so with a rounded low back and then from a slight squat with a straight back. Set the bag down on the other side with a dynamic movement, and then repeat the sequence from the other side.

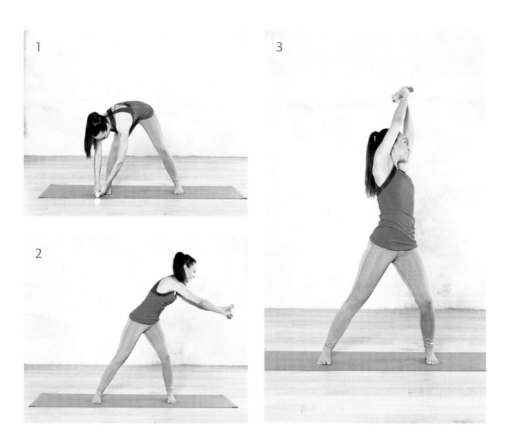

Sky toss

Tool: swing weight or hand weight

1. Stand in a wide straddle position. Place the weight next to your right foot and then pick up the weight with both hands.

2 and 3. Briskly swing the weight to the left and overhead. As you do so, push off with your right foot and guide the weight in a wide arc to the left and upward. Next work the other side.

Do 3, 5, 7, or 10 repetitions per side; gradually increase.

Tone

1

2

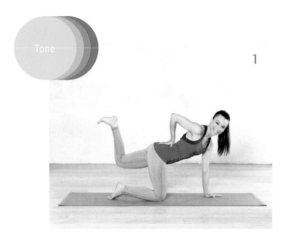
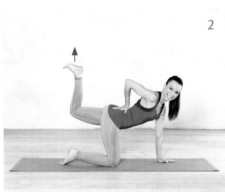

Bouncing foot tray

1. Begin on all fours. Raise your left leg and bend the knee so the lower leg is at a 90° angle to the upper leg. Rest your right palm on your left buttock and if possible look over your shoulder to your left foot. The foot is flexed as though you were balancing a tray on the bottom of your foot.

2. Now bounce the left leg up towards the ceiling. Then switch sides and work the right leg.

Work each side until you have exhausted the muscles.

Bouncing foot tray with ankle weight

Tool: ankle weights

You can increase the exercise intensity by wearing an ankle weight. Tip: Start with the easier version and then do the more intense one.

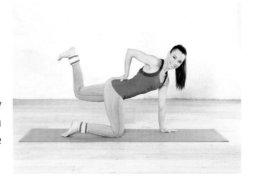

1   2   3

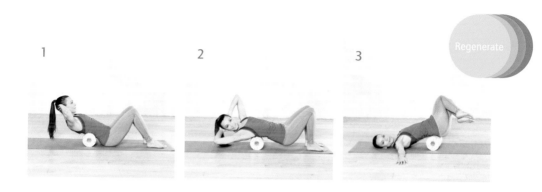

Rolling the back

Tool: large foam roller with smooth surface

1. Lie on your back, plant your feet, and place the roller below your shoulder blades. Cross your hands at the base of the skull; elbows point to the outside. Now firmly press your feet into the floor and slightly lift your pelvis off the floor.

2. Nestle your upper back into the roller in different directions, a little higher, a little to the side, twisting.

3. Now push the roller farther down toward the lumbar spine and rest your upper body on the floor with the arms extended to the sides. Pull your knees into the chest and gently roll your lower back. Turn your head to the right when you let your knees fall to the left, and vice versa. Roll all the way down to the gluteal muscles and back up, similar to a bear rubbing his back on a tree.

Plantar Fascia-Heel Pad-Achilles Tendon Chain

You probably already know how important strong foot muscles are and how bad misalignment of the feet can be. But usually only insiders know that a tough connective tissue layer covers the entire sole of the foot, and that this plantar fascia, among other things, determines the tension in the arch of the foot. The mark of a healthy plantar fascia is its great firmness. If the sole of the foot were flexible like a rubber snake we would move like one, namely we would crawl.

The next outstanding structure that gives us our elastic gait is the Achilles tendon. As we walk, run, skip, and jump, it lengthens and shortens much like a rubber band and facilitates springy jumps like those of a kangaroo. To return to their naturally powerful, elastic tension, our civilized floppy feet that have degenerated due to underuse, and our weak Achilles tendons require targeted strengthening. Over the coming weeks you should patiently build up these elastic structures, and the following exercises will show you how.

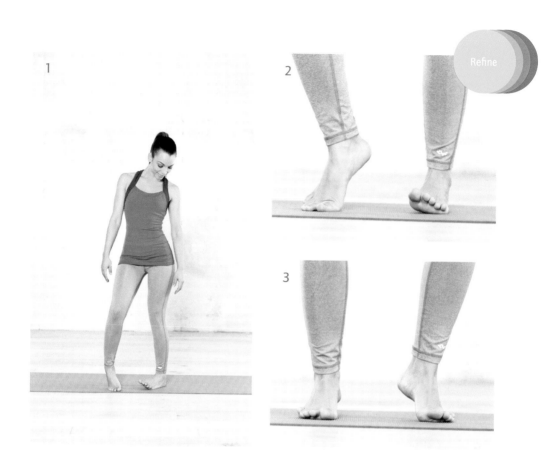

Refine

Foot flow

1, 2, and 3. In a standing position, experiment with small foot movements. As you do so, keep the foot close to the floor. Shift your weight in a fluid motion to the outside of the foot, to the middle of the foot, and then to the inside.

Spread your toes like claws and lift each toe one at a time as though you were trying to lengthen them. Toes three and four will be a challenge. The more small angles and nestling pressure you can create during contact with the floor the more you will stimulate the many plantar fascia receptors searching for sensory news. The reward follows on the heels: Such an active sole makes walking and jumping much more stable and easier.

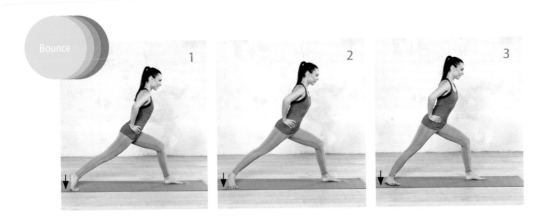

Strengthening the plantar fascia and the Achilles tendon

1. Step forward into a lunge with the left foot. Align the knee over the ankle and extend the right leg so far back that you are pressing the front of that foot firmly into the floor and are able to raise the heel. Hands rest on hips. Now bounce your right heel towards the floor. The impulse originates in the raised heel, which quickly bounces downward. Use the brief contact with the floor to strengthen the Achilles tendon.

2. Change the position of the right leg to stimulate different parts of the Achilles tendon. Plant your foot slightly more to the outside, to the inside, or at a slant.

3. To involve the plantar fascia even more, also lift the toes while bouncing the Achilles tendon. Next switch legs to work the left leg.

Do 3, 5, 7, or 10 repetitions per variation; gradually increase.

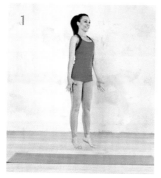
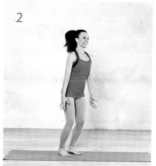
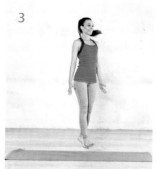

Kangaroo jump

1 and 2. Tighten your catsuit and maintain that whole-body tension during all elastic jumps. Jump into the air with both legs and land with your legs nearly extended. Become a bouncing rubber ball. Here the intensity of your body tension, the only slightly bent knees, and the brief contact with the floor determine whether you are working the elastic Achilles tendon and leg fascia or the muscles.

3. Vary your jumps by landing and jumping with both legs in different foot positions.

Do 3, 5, 7, or 10 jumps; gradually increase.

High-knee skips

Skip in place from one leg to the other and alternate raising the knees. As you do so, open your hands and spread your fingers, bend the elbows, and pump the arms.

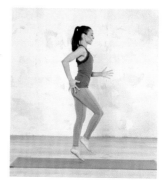

Do 10 to 15 jumps; gradually increase.

Tone

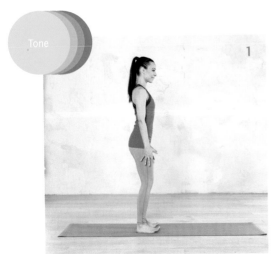
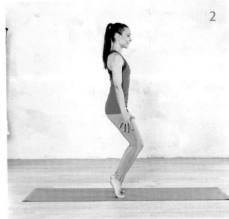

Foot seesaw

1. In a standing position, rock from the heel to the ball of the foot with both feet. The emphasis is on the forward-and-up motion impulse. Stay on the balls of the feet, hold this position, and add additional up-and-down mini bounces originating in the instep.

2. Vary the exercise by rocking onto your toes. This exercise strengthens the Achilles tendon's aponeurosis that is essential for elastic bounces and jumps. Skip this exercise if you prefer slender calves, and move on to the next one. Otherwise hold this position until the muscles are exhausted. This exercise is a must for fallen arches and flat feet!

Continue the exercise until the muscles are exhausted.

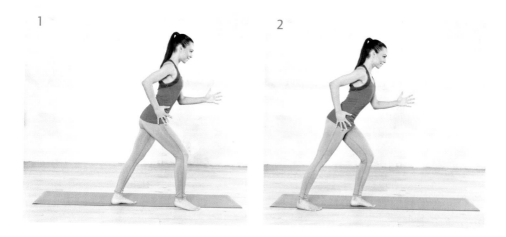

Tooth and claw

1. Stand with your legs astride and the right leg in front.

2. Drag your left foot backward with a powerful dynamic motion as though you were trying to make a deep furrow in the ground. As you do so, expose your teeth and claws. The tooth-and-claw principle marks the gripping vitalization. Add a power sound ("huh" or "heh") as you drag the foot backward. Next slide the right foot back into starting position and then drag it backward again with teeth and claws exposed. Switch sides and work the left foot.

Continue the exercise until the muscles are exhausted.

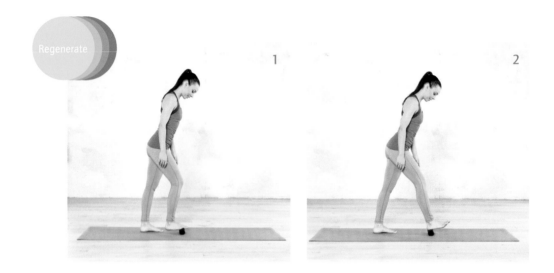

Regenerate

Rolling the plantar fascia

Tool: mini foam roller (tennis ball as an alternative)

1. Place the mini roller under the ball of the right foot. Shift your bodyweight to the right foot and firmly push the roller along the bottom of the foot toward the heel.

2. Start at the ball of the foot behind the big toe and roll your first track towards the heel. Next roll the second track from the heel to the second toe. From there roll the third track back to the heel. Roll a total of five tracks, covering the entire plantar fascia all the way to the little toe.

Tip: two rolling qualities

The first version is rolling to tone. Here the pressure should be firm and the rolling pace brisk to increase tension in the plantar fascia or the Achilles tendon.

The second version stimulates the hydrating and regenerating processes. The rolling pace should therefore be slow and steady.

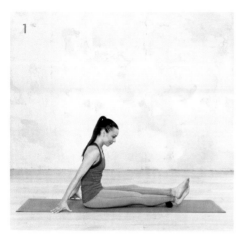 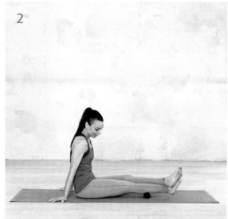

Rolling the Achilles tendon

Tool: mini foam roller

1. Sit with your legs extended and your hands propped behind your body. Now cross the left leg over the right and place the foam roller below the right leg at the heel.

2. Now roll with firm and steady pressure from the heel to just below the knee. As you do so, slightly push off the floor with your hands so the roller can roll more easily along the calf. Roll multiple tracks back and forth.

Everyday exercise: step antelope

Stair steps are an excellent training tool for the fascia of your legs. Bounce up and down the stairs with a spring in your step. As you do so, occasionally vary your foot position and stride. For instance, you can plant your feet slightly sideways, take two steps at once, or jump like a kangaroo with both feet at once as you go up the stairs. Guaranteed fun!

Foot Arch-Adductors-Pelvic Floor Chain

This segment focuses on an important stabilizing chain that is interconnected from the feet—particularly the longitudinal arch of the foot—to the adductors, and all the way to the front area of the pelvic floor.

Strengthening this chain has a far-reaching effect as it greatly contributes to an upright posture. Whether we slump or stand up tall largely depends on the tension of the pelvic floor that is stretched across the pelvis similar to an elastic trampoline whose edges are bent upward. In past years, we specifically emphasized the strengthening of muscles in pelvic floor exercises, but the loss of tension depends significantly on fibrosis, meaning the collagen fibers grow brittle and stick together. This results in a loss of flexibility and elastic resistance. The tightly stretched trampoline turns into a saggy hammock. Today, armed with this increased knowledge and an innovative approach, we train differently to specifically strengthen the fascial elastic parts of the pelvic floor.

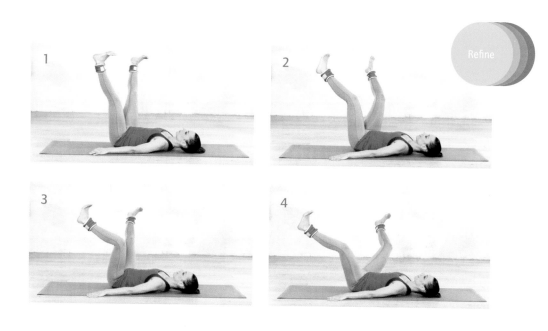

Adductors and waking up the pelvic floor

Tool: ankle weights

1. Fasten the ankle weights around your ankles and lie on your back with arms alongside the body. Make sure that your lower back rests on the floor and your back is not arched. Place your legs in a straddle position, but not too far apart. The focus is less on stretching the inside of the legs but rather more on switching on your awareness all the way into the pelvic floor.

2, 3 and 4. Slightly bend your knees and twist your legs alternately to the inside and outside in a fluid motion while also widening your legs gently and in a controlled manner. In places where your legs want to just give way, move more slowly and even more fluidly and bring these blind spots back into your body awareness.

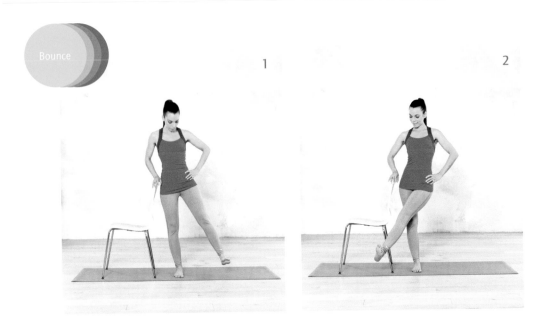

Bounce

1

2

Adductor kick (easy)

1 and 2. Stand next to a chair with your legs hip-width apart. Now begin by swinging the left leg across the right leg in front of the body with your foot flexed. Stabilize your stance by lightly leaning on the chair. Switch sides and work the other leg.

Do 3, 5, 7, or 10 repetitions per side; gradually increase.

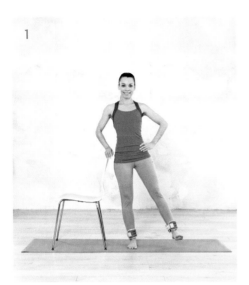

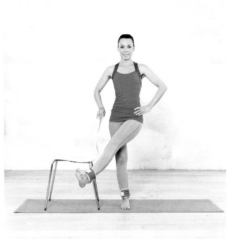

Adductor kick with ankle weights (advanced)

Tool: ankle weights

1 and 2. You can intensify the exercise by wearing ankle weights. Doing so will load the collagen chain at the inside of the leg even more.

Variation:

You can also work with a bolster or a medicine ball and kick it away with your adductor leg swing, a plus when tightening this chain.

Do 3, 5, 7, or 10 repetitions per side; gradually increase.

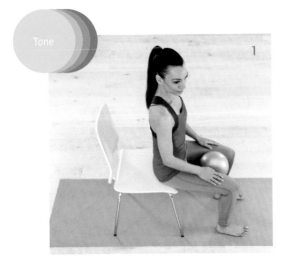
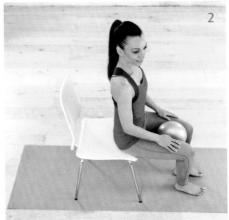

Adductor tightener (easy)

Tool: Overball or mini exercise ball (a rolled up towel as an alternative)

Sit on the front edge of a chair. As you do so, feel your sit bones, which means there is no pressure on your tailbone and you have the correct posture.

1. Now wedge the ball between your thighs and squeeze the ball with your legs in a bouncing motion. Make a sharp power sound ("tz") during each release phase.

2. Finish the exercise by steadily and firmly squeezing the ball and then bouncing into this final position with 15 quick mini bounces.

Continue the exercise until the muscles are exhausted.

1   2

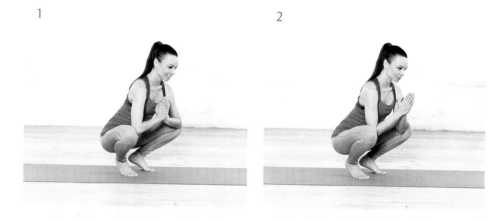

Adductor tightener (intermediate)

1. Sink into a deep squat and lift your heels off the floor. Place your palms together in prayer hands and squeeze your forearms between your thighs.

2. Now build up tension by pressing the inner thighs into the arms; palms continue to press together. Bounce with your inner thighs against the resistance of the arms. The upper-thigh movements are small and focused.

Continue the exercise until the muscles are exhausted.

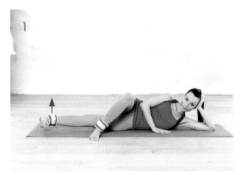 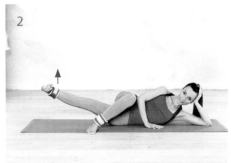

Adductor tightener with ankle weights (advanced)

Tool: ankle weights

1. You will use ankle weights for this exercise. Lie on your left side and support your head with your left hand. You can rest the right arm in front of the body. The left leg is extended and the right foot is planted in front of the left leg. Now lift your left leg a couple inches off the floor, flex the foot, and do little mini bounces toward the ceiling.

2. Next lift the leg a little higher and intensify the exercise with 10 additional mini bounces.

Tip: Slightly vary the foot position of the bouncing leg to work as many areas within the network as possible. Switch sides and then work the right leg.

Work each side until the muscles are exhausted.

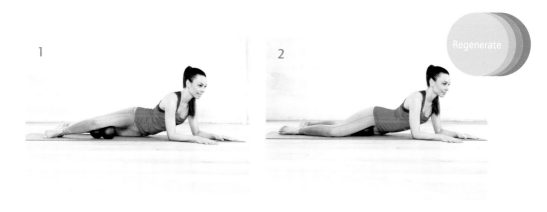

Rolling the inside leg

Tool: large foam roller with smooth surface or large Duoball

1. Lie on your stomach, resting on your forearms. Bend the right knee and place the Duoball above the knee under your thigh. Now roll the inside of the thigh up to the hip joint and back again with slow melting pressure.

2. The Duoball will allow you to roll a little more to the inside and higher, up to the pubic branch. The pubic branch is the bony connection between the pubis in front and the ischium in back. Here you already reach the area of the pelvic floor.

Everyday exercise: purse squeeze

If you commute by train, bus, or subway, you can easily get in a little strengthening adductor-pelvic floor unit. Place your purse between your knees and slowly squeeze it in a bouncing motion. I am sure no one will notice what you are doing, and your pelvic floor will thank you!

Cellulite Special: The Fascia Lata

As soon as they hear the phrase *connective tissue*, many women immediately think cellulite.

They do so in connection with their daily battles with the hated thighs, with brush massages, cold fusions, and the use of various expensive cosmetics touted by the cosmetics industry. No matter which impressive, seemingly scientific formula graces the jar, to date there is no credible proof that anti-cellulite products permanently tighten connective tissue. No ingenious recipe for a crème, lotion, or tincture can replace what exercise can accomplish.

So far, there is no scientific study on fascia training with respect to improving tissue affected by cellulite. Nevertheless, based on findings from fascia research, we can offer some definite advice here regarding which types of treatments and exercise will specifically and permanently strengthen the collagen structures.

Connective tissue, cellulite, and firm thighs

Cellulite shows up wherever fat deposits below the skin and weak connective tissue meet. With respect to collagen fibers, weak means too soft and therefore not providing sufficient resistance and support. When it comes to cellulite, genetic predisposition plays an important role. The effects of estrogen also increase tissue elasticity. Women are therefore more likely than men to develop the so-called mattress phenomenon.

Furthermore the collagen architecture in women is less lattice-like and less cross-linked in different directions, and the arrangement of collagen fibrils—the finest collagen fibers—is more wide-meshed. This causes the distances between individual segments to increase, allowing bulky accumulations of fat cells to cluster there. When the connective tissue in the sheath surrounding the thighs—the fascia lata—is too soft and stretchy, larger fat pads on the thighs create unsightly dents.

But in female athletes and women with firmer connective tissue, the dense and resistant membrane on the outside of the thigh, the tractus iliotiibialis, or the IT band for short, in particular counteracts this with its sturdy structure. In this dense and strong connective tissue network, the collagen meshes are interwoven in a lattice pattern and fat cells are contained in a toned net by many close-meshed segments.

These women have the longed-for firm thighs, but tend to be plagued by so-called runner's knee, a type of overloading of the IT band, which gets matted and has too much tension on it. Cellulite is not usually a problem for female athletes. Conclusion: A strong IT band and cellulite are mutually exclusive.

The success formula to tighten your thighs

We also use our success formula when it comes to tightening the thighs. By applying the findings listed above, we plunge head first into strengthening the fascia lata, and that puts the two active aspects of training front and center: elastic bouncing and tightening muscles.

The IT band together with the plantar fascia and Achilles tendon serve as the master fascia for a two-legged gait via a collagenous bond. In a crawling infant, the outside of the thigh is still unformed and the fascia is soft. It only begins to get strong when dealing with gravity while standing, running, and jumping. A strong IT band that extends out from the fascia lata specifically at the outside of the thigh allows us to balance on one leg, an essential requirement for walking on two legs and for the human long-distance runner.

But "Use it or lose it" is the implacable law of connective tissue dynamics. Sitting around for hours on end, regardless of the important career-related reasons, comes at a price. It is quite simple: Dynamic, bouncing leg movements and muscle toning determine saggy or tight thighs. This is the reason we capitalized on these two elements in the cellulite program and work on them more extensively than the others. If you want firm thighs, get out of your comfort zone and into running, skipping, and jumping! It tightens the thighs and is also lots of fun.

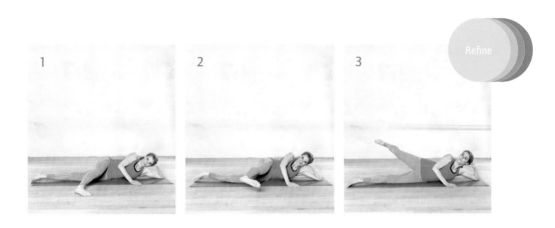

Tentacle leg

1. Lie on your left side and rest your head in your left hand. You can support yourself with the right hand in front of the body. The left leg is an extension of the upper body, the right leg is extended forward at a right angle. Press the right foot into the floor so the big toe, the small toes, and the outside of the heel are anchored to the floor. The foot should practically suction itself to the floor with those three points of contact while tightening the entire length of the outer thigh.

2. Lift your right leg and slightly bend the knee without losing basic tension. Now start to push the leg forward and back with the foot initiating the movement. Imagine you are trying to push away an imaginary cardboard wall.

3. After you push the leg back, stretch a little farther, first through the heel and then every individual toe. Find new angles and positions in fluid motion and move the leg slightly up and down, similar to an octopus' tentacle exploring its surroundings. Switch sides and work the other leg.

Bounce

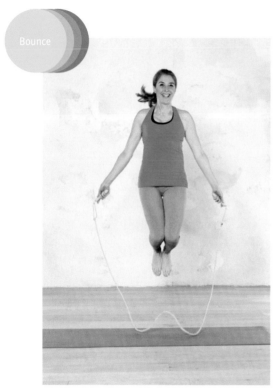

Jumping rope

Tool: jump rope

There is nothing better! Jumping rope is the ideal exercise for cultivating elastic, strong collagen fibers. So are other jumping games like, for instance, hopscotch where the object of the game is to jump into squares drawn with chalk, preferably on one leg.

If you haven't jumped rope since you were a child, it may take a while to regain that hand, wrist, and leg coordination. But it is well worth practicing because you can take a jump rope anywhere and use it in versatile ways, as an invigorating interlude at the park or as a dynamic insertion into your jogging routine. The healthy side effect is that firm thighs are accompanied by improved circulation and a cheerful mood.

You can find source information for suitable jump ropes as well as a hopscotch mat from the area of functional fitness on page 176. Plan on jumping rope a minimum of 10 minutes twice a week. However, to permanently build elastic and strong collagen fibers, you should always take at least a 48-hour break between dynamic bouncing units.

Kangaroo jump (advanced)

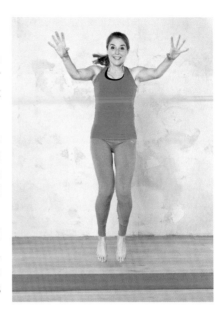

You are already familiar with the easy version of the kangaroo jump from the previous chapter (see page 137). Repeat that exercise to start and then switch to the more advanced version.

Jump into the air with both legs and land with your legs nearly extended. Turn into a bouncing rubber ball. The intensity of the body tension and the brief contact with the floor are essential to train the elastic structures.

In the advanced version, you jump forward and back three times with both legs. As you do so, keep your arms extended forward and maintain tension throughout the body, literally to the tips of your hair.

Do 3, 5, 7, or 10 jumps per version; gradually increase.

Skip (advanced)

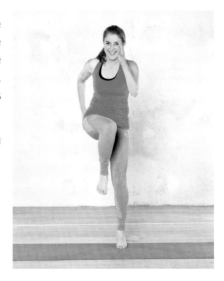

You are already familiar with this basic exercise as well (see page 137), but now you will increase the intensity. Skip in place from one leg to the other, raising alternating knees as you do so. Tighten your catsuit by spreading your hands and fingers wide and pumping the arms.

Do 10 to 15 jumps at top speed. Jumps follow in quick succession.

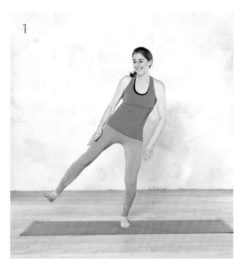
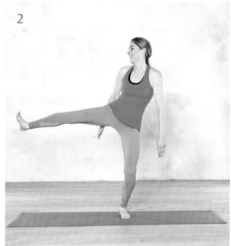

Bouncing single-leg kick

1 and 2. Shift your weight to your left leg and keep hopping. The heel of the left foot remains lifted and you land only on the ball of the foot. The right leg makes small, sharp kicks to the side, downward and as high as possible. Then switch to the right leg and kick with the left.

Do 3, 5, 7, or 10 repetitions per side; gradually increase.

Tips for jumping and running workouts

Week 1: If you have not practiced bouncing jumps for a long time, start with a short intensive exercise sequence. Begin with 2 minutes of jumping rope, then take a 30-second break followed by the easy kangaroo jump and the bouncing single-leg kick.

Week 2: The exercise sequence remains the same, but now you wait until after the single-leg kick to take a break. Then repeat the entire exercise sequence. Ideally you will do this format three times a week.

Week 3: The following week you increase the volume a little and add the skip into your exercise program. Doing a third set of the entire exercise sequence will add intensity.

Week 4: This week we will add jogging to the training plan. Practice the familiar exercise sequence and in addition go for a run twice a week. Ten minutes are enough, but build in short sprints. Start with 5-step sprints, then jog a few steps, then add two more short sprints. Increase the sprints to 25 steps over the coming weeks and build two sprints into each of your runs.

Make your training versatile! Mix up the elastic bouncing exercises to keep the workouts interesting and as a way to add new stimuli for collagen synthesis. Work on your jumping and running elements for at least 10 minutes on the same three days of the week for three months. The shape of your thighs will not improve instantly, but you can expect a definite noticeable and visibly firmer contour within this window of time.

This is important for building collagen fibers with a healthy lattice-like structure long-term: The regeneration period of 48 hours between loading phases must be observed!

Tone

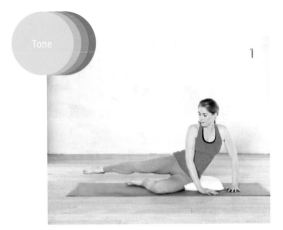

1

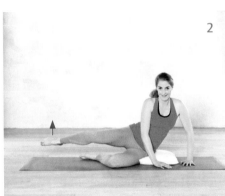

2

Thigh tightener (easy)

Start the following thigh-tightening exercises with the easier versions, which are already quite challenging, and increase the intensity over the coming weeks. Allow yourself some variety! You have different tools at your disposal to do so.

1. Sit on your left side with the left knee bent in front of the body and the right leg extended. You can support the pelvis with a pillow as shown in the photo. Support your upper body with your arms to make it a little easier. Drop the shoulders and reach up with the crown of the head.

2. Now lift the right leg, bend the knee, and make small bouncing movements toward the ceiling. Switch sides and work the left leg.

Work each side until the muscles are exhausted.

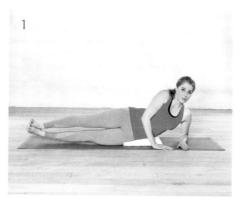 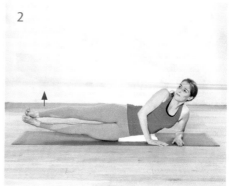

Thigh tightener (intermediate)

1. Remain on your side and extend both legs.

2. Now bounce both extended legs towards the ceiling. You can rest your left forearm on the floor; place the right hand in front of the body for support. Here you are working with a long lever, which is quite challenging and only suitable for women who can remain stable in this position. Next switch sides.

Work each side until the muscles are exhausted.

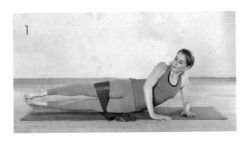
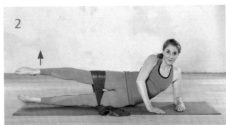
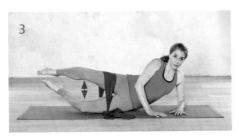
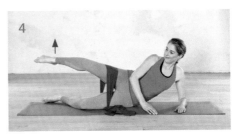

Thigh tightener with resistance band (advanced)

Tool: resistance band

1 and 2. Firmly tie the resistance band around your legs above the knees. Lie on your side and support yourself with your arms as before. Now lift both legs off the floor and bounce against the band's resistance while maintaining tension on the band.

3. Now bend the knees slightly and work against the band's resistance by opening your legs with a bouncing movement.

4. The easier beginner version: The left leg remains on the floor and you bounce upward with only the right leg. Next switch sides.

Do each version and work each side until the muscles are exhausted.

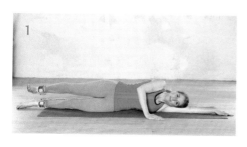
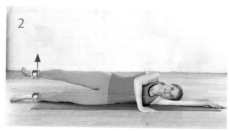
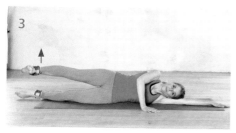
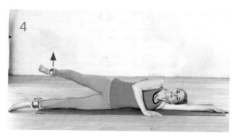

Thigh tightener with ankle weights (advanced)

Tools: ankle weights

1 and 2. Strap on the ankle weights. Lie on your left side and rest your head on the extended left arm. If necessary, you can support yourself with your right hand in front of the body. Legs are extended. Now lift the right leg and bounce towards the ceiling.

3. Vary the exercise by moving the right leg forward and turning the foot slightly inward, and bounce the leg in this position.

4. Now move the right leg slightly behind the body and turn the foot slightly outward, and bounce the leg in this position. Switch sides and then work the left leg.

Work each side until the muscles are exhausted.

Please note: Tighten your catsuit from the crown of the head down to the toes.

Add-on: high-intensity positions

As soon as you have mastered the basic exercises you will be ready to challenge yourself with the following advanced exercises and combinations. Here the fascial corset is also activated—primarily in the deep abdominal muscles and pelvic region—to tighten the thighs. These positions require strength, coordination, and stability that you will initially build up with the above exercises. We now expand the stabilizing positions via the fascia component and purposefully build in mini bounces. That makes for a super-tightening combination!

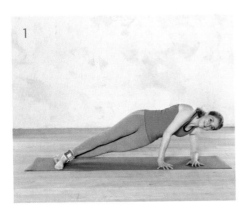
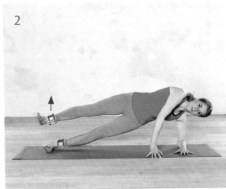

Thigh tightener (very advanced)

Tool: ankle weights

1. Lie on your side and extend both legs. Tighten your fascial corset and push the body off the floor with the left leg, which is tightened all the way to the toes. Use the arms for support.

2. The left leg remains long and stable and the right leg now bounces upward. Hold this position and now also bounce the right leg forward and backward. Occasionally vary the foot position. Switch sides and work the left leg.

Work each side until the muscles are exhausted.

Thigh and pelvis-tightening combination exercise

Tool: ankle weights

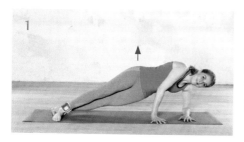

1. Lie on your left side and extend the legs. Tighten your fascial corset and then push the body off the floor with the left leg, which is tightened all the way to the toes. The arms support and stabilize the position. Now do pelvic bounces toward the ceiling.

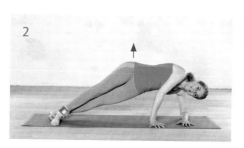

2. For more intensity, lift the pelvis a little higher and bounce from this position.

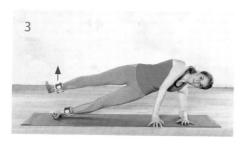

3. Hold your pelvis in place and start to bounce with the right leg to tighten the thigh. Also do all the variations and position changes in front of and behind the body. Add the ankle weights for an additional challenge. Switch sides and then work the left leg.

Work each side and do each variation until the muscles are exhausted.

Regenerate

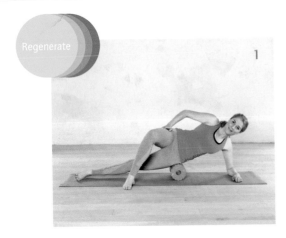
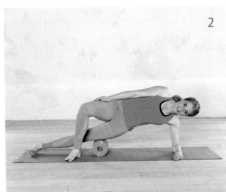

Rolling the outer thigh

Tool: large foam roller with corrugated surface

The corrugated foam roller is particularly well-suited for cellulite treatments because the added pressure from the individual points increases the stimulation of the collagen tissue. If this is too painful at first, start with a smooth foam roller instead. In this case, it is better to increase the treatment intensity over time. You are already familiar with the following exercise from the basic fascia training exercises (see page 90).

Regular rolling of the thighs is essential to the successful treatment of cellulite. In this case, we again use two different qualities of rolling and thereby achieve different effects. We use slow rolling to squeeze out accumulated water and relieve congestion and to stimulate the fluid dynamics within the tissue. The fast and vigorous rolling is used to tone and strengthen the tissue. In both cases, we roll not just in one direction, but rather in as many directions as possible. Combine these two qualities in one rolling session.

1 and 2. Begin by slowly rolling each side of the thigh for 3 to 5 minutes, take a 30-second rehydration break, and then roll fast and vigorously for 2 minutes. You can also build rolling into your workout-free regeneration phase, but definitely work with the roller before and after training units.

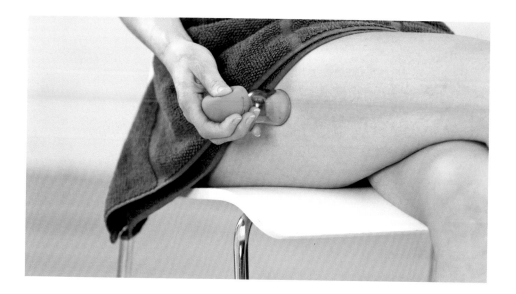

Connective tissue massage for thighs

Tool: Cupping glass

To tighten connective tissue, supplement rolling with a cupping massage, meaning rolling one day and cupping the next day. As with rolling, the same rule applies for cupping: Slowly and vigorously work the outer thigh in lots of different directions.

Which sports have a firming effect on cellulite?

Choose an athletic activity that includes running, jumping, skipping, and kicking. Ball sports like volleyball, team handball, or basketball are good choices.

The importance of running regularly—and we mean running, not power walking—has already been mentioned. Build brief sprints into your running routine like, for instance, three sets of five sprint steps and then return to a jog. If you enjoy dancing, you can take a class like Afro dance, modern dance, or something similar. These types of dances include lots of jumping and skipping.

Many martial arts—such as kung fu, tae kwon do, or karate—include fascial jumps and kicks in addition to the strength and coordination exercises. Using the stepper at your fitness facility is a good alternative, or you can get creative and fearlessly use stairs, a curb on the street, or a low wall at a park for your bouncing fascial purpose. Swimming is definitely healthy but water lacks the important elastic rebound stimulation for the legs that is so important for the anti-cellulite program. You could add a bouncing thigh-tightening unit to your aquatic program by doing a 5- to 10-minute run or jump rope unit prior to your pool workout.

If you are devoted to practicing qigong, yoga, or Pilates, it is important to supplement these valuable exercise programs specifically with elastic jumps to tighten the connective tissue of the thighs.

Everyday exercise: stair antelope special

Forgo using escalators and elevators! Always! Instead, bound up and down the stairs like the previously described stair antelope. Light on your feet, quietly and quickly up and down. Occasionally vary your foot position and stride. Twice a week, build in a special variation and take two or three steps at once going up. This particularly strengthens the thighs and also tightens the buttocks. Carrying a (not too heavy) backpack or purse as you do so gives you the ultimate training advantage.

The Building-Block Principle

Here are a few suggestions for exercise sequences to serve as an incentive for your own workouts. You can set priorities based on which weak areas you identified with the self-test (see page 43) and which parts of the body you would like to emphasize and specifically tighten. The individual sequences can be combined and individual building blocks can of course be substituted with other exercises.

Training sequence: toned arms and a firm chest

Chest opener (see page 113)

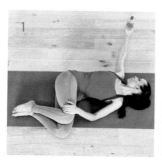 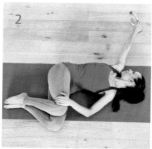 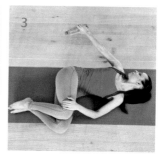

Power arms (see page 106)

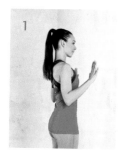 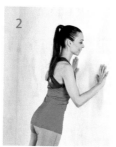 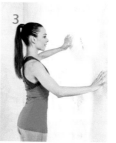 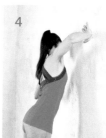

Arm catapult (see page 114)

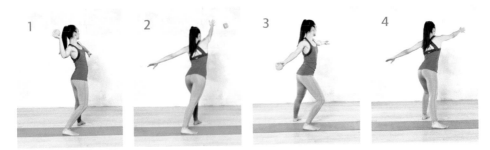

Triceps tightener (see page 108)

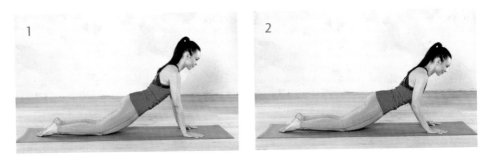

Chest tightener with hand weight (see page 118)

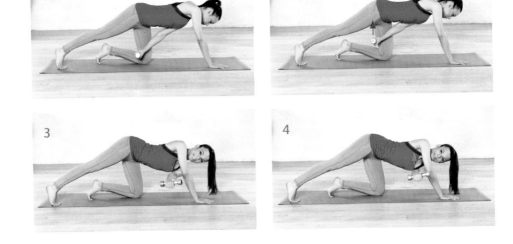

Deltoid tightener (see page 110)

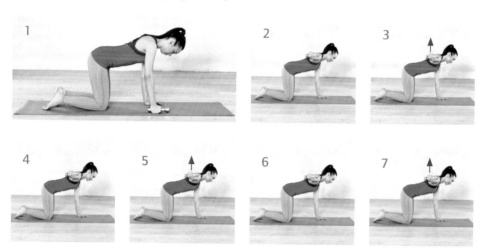

Connective tissue massage for the chest (see page 119)

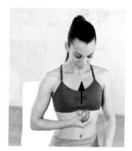

Rolling the arm (see page 111)

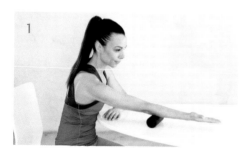
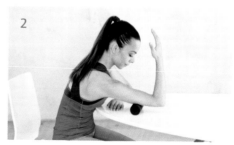

Training sequence: toned core and pelvic floor

Activating the core network (see page 121)

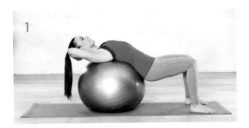 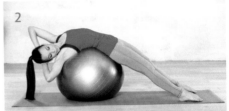

Frog jump (see page 130)

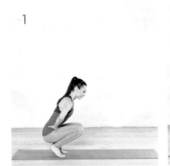 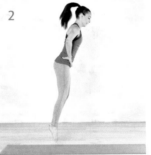 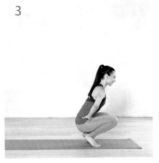

Power throw (see page 123)

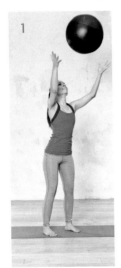 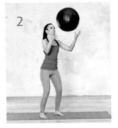 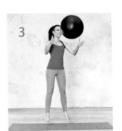 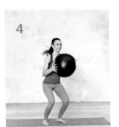

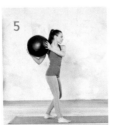 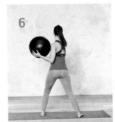 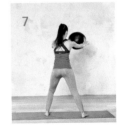

Adductor kick (easy) (see page 144)

1

2

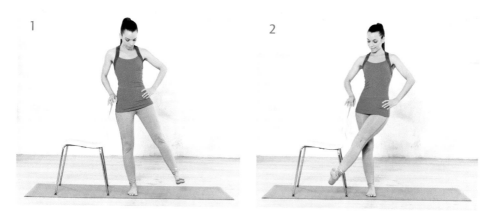

Tightening all of the abdominal muscles (see page 125)

1

2

3

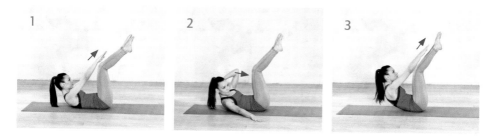

Foot seesaw (see page 138)

1

2

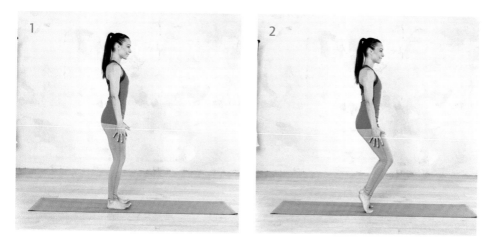

Tightening the waist (advanced) (see page 126)

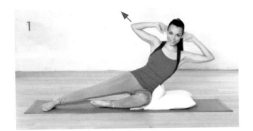 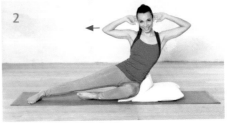

Abdominal connective tissue massage (see page 127)

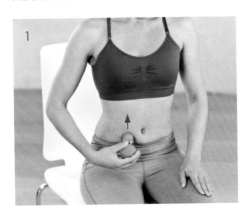 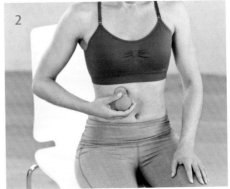

Rolling the inside leg (see page 149)

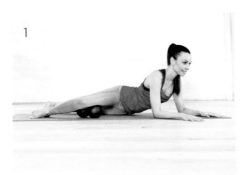 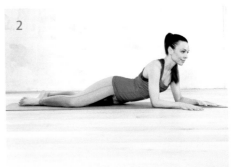

Training sequence: anti-cellulite program and firm thighs

Tentacle leg (see page 153)

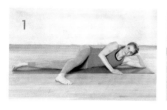 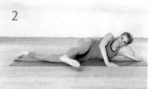 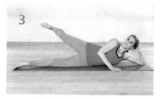

High-knee skips (see page 137)   Kangaroo jump (see page 137)

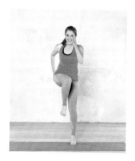 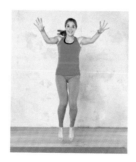

Bouncing single-leg kick (see page 156)

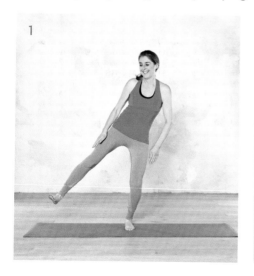 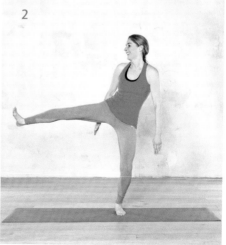

Easy version

Thigh tightener with ankle weights (advanced) (see page 161)

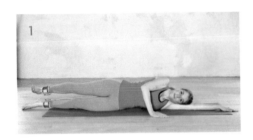
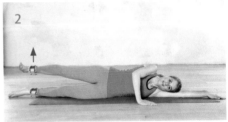
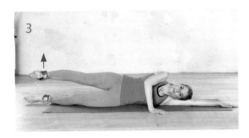
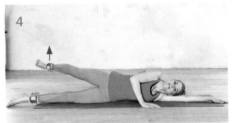

Alternative

Thigh tightener with resistance band (advanced) (see page 160)

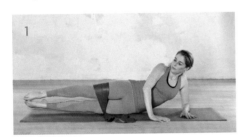
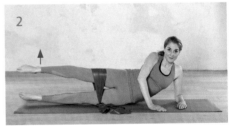
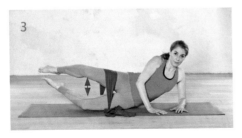
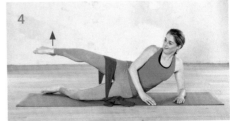

Advanced version

Thigh and pelvis-tightening combination exercise (see page 163)

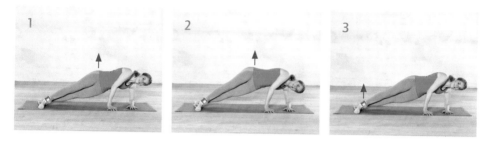

Rolling the outer thigh (see page 164)

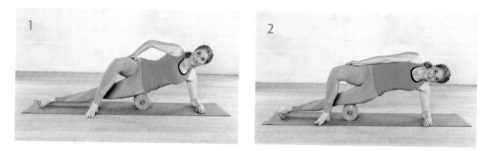

Alternative

Connective tissue massage for thighs (see page 165)

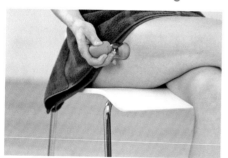

Tools and Tips

Sources for training tools

- Stability ball (ARTZT vitality)
- Exercise mat (ARTZT vitality)
- Mini ball (ARTZT vitality)
- Fascia box

This box was developed in collaboration with the German company ARTZT vitality and provides the perfect basic tool kit for a successful anti-cellulite exercise program. It can be used for various levels of the dynamic jumping elements. It also holds the most important tools for fascia training: a jump rope, a large foam roller, a mini foam roller, a Duoball, and two ankle weights.

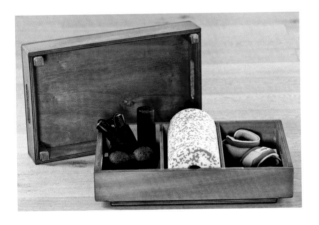 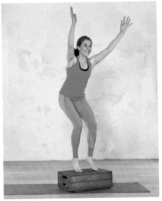

www.artzt-vitality.com

- Resistance band or loop (ARTZT vitality)
- Ankle weights (Thera-Band)
- Hand weights (GYMSTICK™)
- Medicine ball (TOGU)
- Swing weight
- Small weighted ball

- Large smooth foam roller (BLACKROLL®)

- Large groove foam roller (BLACKROLL®)

- Mini foam roller (BLACKROLL®)

- Large Duoball (BLACKROLL®)

- ATX CrossFit ball (ATX®)

- Overball

- Hopscotch mat (adidas Agility Grid)

- Jump rope

- Cupping glass (cupping glass with ball)

Classes, books, and DVDs

- www.fascialnet.com

- www.fascial-fitness.com

Fascial Fitness   *FASCIAL FITNESS*

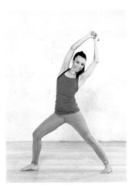

- Certified Fascial Fitness instructor training up to master trainer level

- Continuing training in fascial toning, the new program to tighten connective tissue

- Continuing training in fascial pelvic floor training

- The online shop offers many products on the subject of fascia, such as books and DVDs

Acknowledgments

A heartfelt thank-you to all the wonderful people—many of whom are not listed here—who contributed to the creation of this book. My special thanks to:

Amiena Zylla who, even after long photo shoots, still lit up the camera with her cheerful smile.

Sarah Gast, who committed herself to this project with tenacious kindness from the conception to the execution of countless practical details.

Karin Hertzer who, as co-author, dove into the complex subject of the fascia with enthusiasm and used her competent know-how as a journalist to improve the book's format in so many ways.

Waves of gratitude go to Robert Schleip, PhD, who was always on hand with help and advice regardless of time of day or night, for his enthusiasm for sharing his knowledge of all things fascia with inexhaustible energy and overflowing generosity. It is made all the more precious by the fact that Robert is not only my professional partner, but he is also heart's companion who is at my side through ups and downs. Thank you!

Index

Accident 26, 59
Acetylsalicylic acid 73
Adhesions 27, 113, 127
Advanced glycation end products 53
Agus, David 60
Alexander, Robert McNeill 67
Antioxidants 74-75

Back pain, chronic 13, 28, 91
Back pain, fascial 36
Basic positions 99-101
Basics of fascia training 86-99
Belly fat 72
Bouncing, elastic 152, 157
Building-block principle 167-175
Bulk water 49

Cancer 13, 74
Cellulite 8-9, 23, 29, 36, 54, 56, 150-161,
    164-166, 173
Cilia 55
Climbing and moving hand-over-hand 67
Connective tissue, weak 8, 36, 151
Connective tissue, rigid 37
Connective tissue, tighten 41, 83, 97, 150,
    165, 177
Constitution 37, 40
Contusions 36, 43
Creep effect 29
Crosslinks 25, 32
Crossover type 38-41
Crossover test 42-45
Crystallization 53, 77
Cupping massage 55, 103, 119, 127, 165

Davis, Henry Gassett 60
Davis, Irene 67

Diclofenac 73
Dupuytren's contracture 37
Dynamics, fluid 18, 46-47, 49-50, 52-55,
    164

Earlobes 32, 43
Elasticity 22, 29-30, 52, 67, 80, 82, 87,
    97, 151
Endomysium 15-17
Epimysium 15-18, 34
Enzymes 73-74
    Bromelain 73
    Chymotrypsin 73
    Papain 73
    Trypsin 73
Extracellular matrix (ECM) 48, 51

Harmonic movement 14

Fascia lata 19, 23, 150
Fascia profunda 14, 56
Fascia superficialis 14
Fascia chains
    Abdominal network: straight, oblique
    and transverse abdominals 19, 21, 120-
    127
    Chest-biceps chain 19-20, 112-119
    Cellulite special: fascia lata 150-161
    Fascia lata/thigh fascia 19, 23
    Foot arch-adductors-pelvic floor chain
    19, 23, 142-149
    Plantar fascia-heel pad-Achilles tendon
    chain 19, 22, 134-141
    Diagonal lat-glutes muscle chain 19,
    22, 128-133
    Shoulder-elbow chain 19-20, 104-
    111

Fibroblasts 13, 26, 48, 55, 98
Fibrosis 27, 142
Flexibility and the psyche 35
Foam roller 29, 51-52, 54-55, 85, 89-90, 103, 111, 133, 140-141, 149, 164, 176
Foods
  Good 72-76
  Bad 76

Gender-specificity 32
Guimberteau, Jean-Claude 46

Hardening 28-29
Hemar, Edo 65
Heraclitus 46
Hippocrates 33
Hyaluronic acid 51
Hyaluronan 51-52
Hypermobility and pain 36

Inflammation 36, 53, 61, 70-78
Injury 26-27, 52, 59, 67, 72, 75, 82, 94

Janda, Vladimir 39
Jumping and running workouts 157

Kjær, Michael 97

Lack of exercise 15, 24-25, 28, 50
Langevin, Helen 12
Lieberman, Daniel 66-67, 69
Lymphatic drainage 54, 119

Mechano-adaption 60

Mini bounces 93-94, 96, 109, 116, 126, 138, 146, 148, 162
Movement organ 25
Müller-Wohlfahrt, Hans-Wilhelm 25

Nutrition 70-78

Omega-3 fatty acids 76
Operations 26, 28, 35, 58-59
  Back operations 28
Overloading 27, 50, 82, 98, 102, 151
Overweight 36, 72

Performance capacity, athletic 13, 82
Perimysium 15-16
Pollack, Gerald 49

Refinement, sensory 86, 91, 95
Rehydration 54, 72, 89, 164
Release, fascial 86, 89-90, 95
Rolf, Ida 12

Schleip, Robert 8, 13, 15, 19, 26-28, 32, 34-38, 40, 49-50, 52-53, 59-62, 64-65, 68-70, 77, 178
Scoliosis 36, 44
Stecco, Carla 12, 17, 52
Still, Andrew Taylor 12-13
Stress 13, 25, 27-28, 33, 53, 59, 78, 86
Stretching, fascial 86, 93
Stretching, melting 29, 60, 93-95
Structured water 49-50
Sugar 73, 75-77

Temple dancer type 31-43, 61, 95, 103
  Advantages, biological 34-35
  Disadvantages, biological 36
  Test 42-44

Throwing and hurling 69
Tongue/frenulum 32, 43
Toning 8, 20, 54, 68, 88, 95-97, 99, 102-103, 108, 116, 120, 122, 124, 132, 138, 146, 152, 158

Tools 83-85, 176-177
Training recommendations 102-103
Traumatic events 59

Underloading 27, 70, 98

Viking type 31, 33, 37, 39, 45, 60, 87, 95, 113
Viscoelasticity 29
Viscosity 29
Vitamins 74

Walking/running 18, 59, 66, 87, 135
    Walking barefoot 66-67
Water 14, 15, 18, 29, 46-57, 72, 90
Water accumulation 164
Wolff's law 60
Wound healing 26-27, 44, 71, 73

Yoga 29, 31-34, 38, 59, 69, 166

Credits

Photos:
Lisa Martin, Renate Forster

Hair & makeup:
Nilgün Konya

Models:
Amiena Zylla, Divo Mueller

All additional photos:
P. 15 (left), 30, 49, 64, 77, 84 (ATX CrossFit ball), 86 Adobe Stock
P. 15 (right), 16, 25 fascialnet.com
P. 17 Elsevier: (Purslow, PP (2005): Intramuscular connective tissue and its role in meat quality.
In: Meat Science 70 (3): 435–447)
P. 28 Springer Science and Business Media: (Järvinen, TAH (2002): Organization and distribution of intramuscular connective tissue in normal and immobilized skeletal muscles. In: Journal of Muscle Research and Cell Motility 23 (3))
P. 47 Dr. Jean Claude Guimberteau
P. 84 (large stability ball), 85 (overball) ARTZT vitality

Illustrations:
P. 20-24 Nadine Schurr (source material: Fascial Fitness Association Divo Mueller)
P. 31 courtesy of Robert Schleip, PhD, (source material: Reeves, ND, Narici, MV, Maganaris, CN (2006): Myotendinous Plasticity to Ageing and Resistance Exercise in Humans. In: Experimental Physiology 91(3): 483–498)
P. 34, 42, 43 Südwest Verlag, a Random House, Inc. company (source material: Schleip, Robert (2014): Faszien-Fitness, Riva)
P. 44, 45, 51, 55, 87 courtesy of Robert Schleip, PhD, (source material: Kawakami, Y, Muraoka, T, Ito, S, Kaneshisa, H, Fukunaga, T (2002): In Vivo Muscle Fibre Behaviour during Countermovement Exercisen in Humans Reveals a Significant Role for Tendon Elasticity. In: The Journal of Physiology 540 (2): 635-646)
P. 48, 98 fascialnet.com
P. 53 Annika Naas (source material: Adobe Stock)

Editing: Anne Rumery
Layout: Annika Naas
Typesetting: zerosoft
Cover design: Sannah Inderelst

MORE ON FITNESS

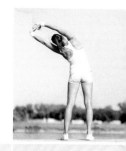

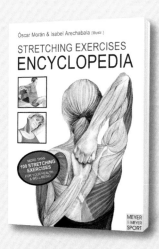

Óscar Morán (author)
Isabel Arechabala (illustrations)

STRETCHING EXERCISES ENCYCLOPEDIA

This book offers a general theory of muscle stretching. Anatomical illustrations explain the different muscle groups involved in the exercises. Furthermore, each exercise includes information about the movement one needs to perform, the posture that one must adopt, common mistakes that should be avoided, the principal and secondary muscles worked with this exercise, as well as a series of very useful tips and advice. Any athlete will realize how regular stretching can improve their physical body shape and their quality of life.

2nd edition
240 p., color, paperback,
265 illustrations,
8 1/4" x 11 1/2"
ISBN: 9781841263519
$ 19.95 US

All information subject to change © Adobe Stock

MEYER & MEYER Sport
Von-Coels-Str. 390
52080 Aachen
Germany

Phone   +49 02 41 - 9 58 10 - 13
Fax   +49 02 41 - 9 58 10 - 10
E-Mail   sales@m-m-sports.com
Website www.m-m-sports.com

All books available as E-books.

MEYER
& MEYER
SPORT

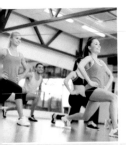

MORE ON FITNESS FROM MEYER & MEYER

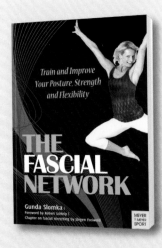

1st edition

280 p., color, paperback,

44 illustrations, 336 photos,

6 1/2" x 9 1/4"

ISBN: 9781782550693

$ 29.95 US

Gunda Slomka

THE FASCIAL NETWORK ENCYCLOPEDIA

TRAIN AND IMPROVE YOUR POSTURE, STRENGTH AND FLEXIBILITY

Fascia have many functions in the human body and this book provides you with everything you need to improve them. The first part contains an overview of the development and anatomy of the connective tissue. This is followed by a practical part with many ideas for your training. Numerous exercises for your fitness and health are included.

All information subject to change © Adobe Stock

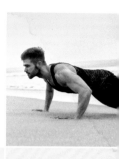

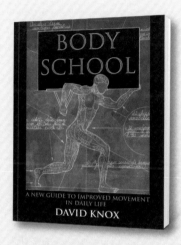

David Knox

BODY SCHOOL

A NEW GUIDE TO IMPROVED
MOVEMENT IN DAILY LIFE

Body School is a user-friendly guide
to making your body last a lifetime.
Whether you are looking to improve your
skills or find a solution to an ongoing
injury or chronic pain, you will find help
in these pages. The information is clearly
laid out, the stretches, exercises, and
therapies easy to understand and easy
to follow.

1st edition

358 p., color, paperback,

64 photos,

7.7" x 10"

ISBN: 9781782550587

$ 34.95 US

All information subject to change © Adobe Stock

MEYER & MEYER Sport
Von-Coels-Str. 390
52080 Aachen
Germany

Phone   +49 02 41 - 9 58 10 - 13
Fax   +49 02 41 - 9 58 10 - 10
E-Mail   sales@m-m-sports.com
Website www.m-m-sports.com

All books available as E-books.

MEYER
& MEYER
SPORT

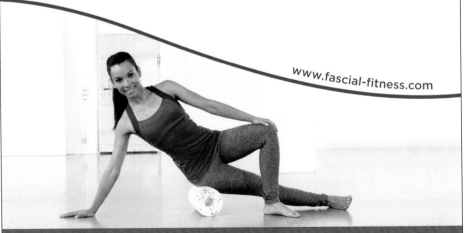

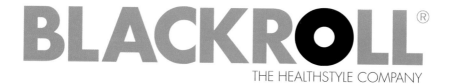
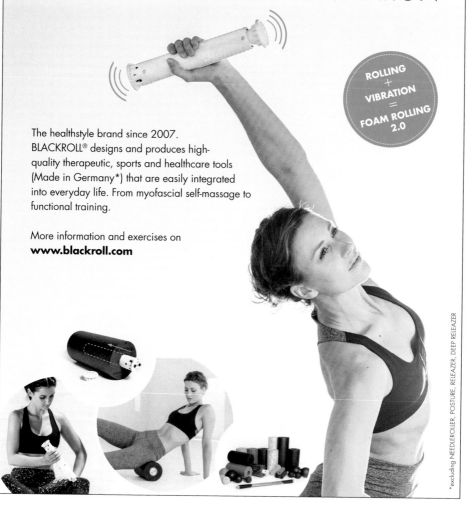

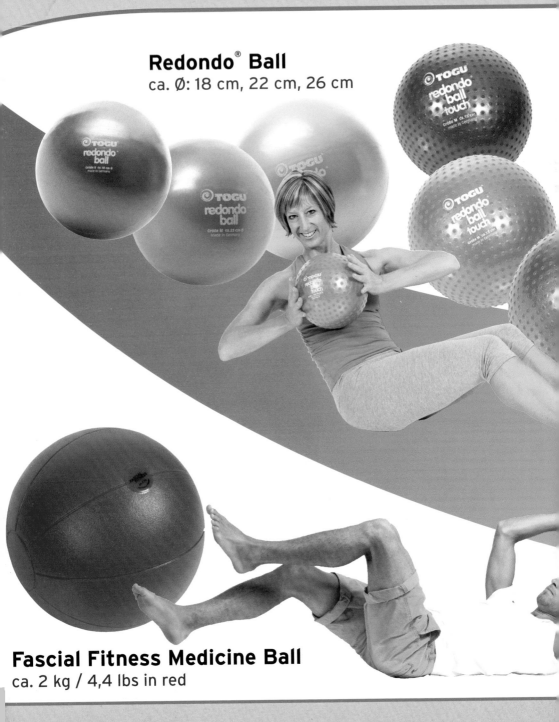

TOGU®

Redondo® Ball
ca. Ø: 18 cm, 22 cm, 26 cm

Fascial Fitness Medicine Ball
ca. 2 kg / 4,4 lbs in red

TOGU GmbH · Atzinger Str. 1 · D-83209 Prien - Bachham · Fon: +49 (0) 80 51 | 90 38 - 0 ·

Ball series
...use
..., foldable and durable
...ferent sizes

...o® Ball touch
...m, 22 cm, 26 cm

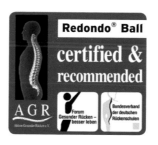
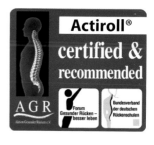

Actiroll®
First air-filled fascia roll
• hardness individually adjustable
• roll and move even on joints

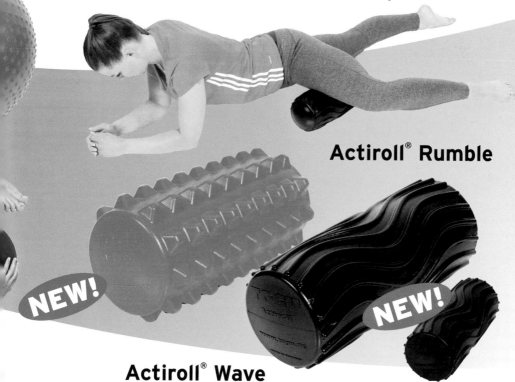

Actiroll® Rumble

NEW!

Actiroll® Wave

NEW!

Actiroll® Wave size „S"

Certified and recommended: Gesunder Rücken – besser leben e.V. and the Bundesverband deutscher Rückenschulen (BdR) e.V.
More infos: www.agr-ev.de

Quality Product — Germany — Made in Germany